Acute Surgery:
The Survival Guide

Edited by

SHELLY GRIFFITHS

MB BS MA (Cantab) MRCS

Radcliffe Publishing

London • New York

Radcliffe Publishing Ltd
33–41 Dallington Street
London
EC1V 0BB
United Kingdom

www.radcliffehealth.com

_____

British Library Cataloguing in Publication Data

A catalogue record for this book is available from the British Library.

ISBN-13: 978 184619 999 8

Designed and typeset by Darkriver Design, Auckland, New Zealand
Printed and bound by Cadmus Communications, USA

Contents

Preface

As a medical student, foundation doctor or surgical trainee, you may find yourself covering a specialty or subspecialty on call in which you have little or no experience. The range of conditions seen can be daunting to the junior trainee trying to come up with a comprehensive management plan (and answering the consultant's questions on the post-take round!). This book is aimed at all juniors who want to be confident in dealing with acute presentations commonly seen in a surgical take. It offers a fail-safe approach to the management of patients in general surgery, vascular surgery, urology, ENT and orthopaedics. As well as these, there are sections on management of commonly seen ward issues and the approach to a trauma patient.

For the most part, this book assumes you have a stable patient – the basic principles of 'ABC' always come first, and only when you are happy with these should you move on to investigating and treating as described in this book. There is also no substitute for a senior review – this is of course what middle-grade doctors and consultants are there for! If you are unsure, ask somebody for help: you should never be criticised for doing this.

This book aims to be the go-to guide that you need to survive a surgical take in style – good luck!

Shelly Griffiths
January 2013

List of contributors

Pratik Roy BSc FRCS (Gen)
Specialist Registrar in General Surgery

Sophie Whelan-Johnson BSc MB BS MRCS
Specialist Registrar in General Surgery

Matthew Stephenson MSc FRCS (Gen)
Specialist Registrar in General Surgery

Elizabeth Bright BMedSci (Hons) MB ChB MRCS
Specialist Registrar in Urology

Helen Teixeira MB BCh MRCS
Core Surgical Trainee

Venkat M Reddy MRCS DOHNS
Specialist Registrar in ENT

Warren O Bennett MA (Oxon) MB BS MRCS DOHNS
ENT Core Surgical Trainee

Benjamin Bradley BSc (Hons) MB BS MRCS
Specialist Registrar in Trauma & Orthopaedics

Al-Amin Kassam BSc (Hons) MB BS MRCS
Specialist Registrar in Trauma & Orthopaedics

Major Thomas König BSc (Hons) MB BS MRCS RAMC
Specialist Registrar in Vascular & Trauma Surgery

Shelly Griffiths MB BS MA (Cantab) MRCS
Core Surgical Trainee

Emma J Noble BA (Oxon) BM BCh MRCS DM
Specialist Registrar in General Surgery

List of figures

Chapter 1

GENERAL SURGERY

Pratik Roy and
Sophie Whelan-Johnson

The acute abdomen

The acute abdomen could be a sign of anything from appendicitis to a ruptured aortic aneurysm, so it's essential to get the basics right, since the patient must be assumed to be unstable and could deteriorate at any point. The most important things to remember are airway, breathing and circulation. As a surgical F2 or CT, forget the old medical student adage of 'History, examination and investigation'. When assessing the patient with an acute abdomen, you can ascertain the important points in the history while simultaneously performing diagnostic and therapeutic manoeuvres such as checking vital signs, making sure an oxygen mask is on the patient, and inserting a cannula and taking blood, including an arterial blood gas (ABG). If the patient is cardiovascularly unstable, it is important to call for senior help at this point, before returning to the patient and ensuring adequate venous access, i.e. two wide-bore cannulae in the antecubital fossae. Remember to take bloods for glucose (in case of pancreatitis) and group and save, as well as the usual urea, electrolytes, amylase, etc. It is always a good idea to obtain an erect chest X-ray and, for most cases, a plain supine abdominal film as well. However, if the patient is very young, pregnant or in the case of suspected appendicitis, then X-rays are not indicated.

Remember that the patient will be in pain. The notion that prescribing strong analgesia will somehow mask the signs is nonsense and will be detrimental to patient care. Paracetamol (1 g qds) should always be given regularly IV, as it has both analgesic and antipyretic effects. Opiate analgesia is almost always required PRN, and sometimes regularly as well. It is good practice to write up naloxone (400 mcg) and a strong anti-emetic such as cyclizine (50 mg tds) or ondansetron (4–8 mg tds).

Adequate fluid resuscitation is vital. Most hospitals have now moved away from using normal saline and dextrose, and prefer using Hartmann's or colloids in the acute setting. Make sure you know your own hospital protocol. Titrate the fluids according to the patient's clinical condition – don't just write up three 8-hourly bags for everyone! To catheterise or not is always a difficult decision. In practice, you will never be told off for catheterising a patient, so err on the side of caution. However, common sense must be used; for stable patients who are perfectly capable of using a jug to record their urine output, a simple fluid balance chart may be enough.

By the time your registrar or consultant reviews the patient, it is helpful to have the relevant blood results and radiology available, but do not delay contacting your seniors simply because results are outstanding if the patient is unwell and likely to need intervention. You should, however, have formulated a working diagnosis when you present the patient to them. Although you may have already decided that the patient warrants further specialist investigation like CT or ultrasound, in most cases these can only be requested after a senior review or by the seniors themselves. However, in obvious cases where patients will require surgery, you can save time by alerting the anaesthetists and theatres. You should not feel pressured into consenting patients for operations, particularly complex laparotomies. However, if you have sufficient experience and feel confident, then you will earn valuable brownie points from your registrar or consultant if you consent the patient and ask your senior colleagues to countersign the consent form.

Be wary of referrals of patients with IBD as an acute abdomen. Exacerbations may present with abdominal pain and diarrhoea, and you will often be asked to rule out a surgical cause of their pain. These patients are normally very complex and the gastroenterologists will want to lead their management.

Right iliac fossa pain

Differential diagnosis of RIF pain:
- appendicitis
- mesenteric adenitis
- Crohn's disease
- UTI
- diverticulitis (including Meckel's).

In women:
- ectopic pregnancy
- ovarian/tubal pathology
- Mittelschmertz.

The commonest general surgical procedure performed is appendicectomy, and so it is not surprising that the commonest referral to the surgical team is for right iliac fossa (RIF) pain. However, there are other causes of RIF pain than appendicitis, most notably ovarian or tubal pathology in females, and Meckel's diverticulitis or small bowel pathology in either sex. Uncommonly in the older population, caecal carcinoma can also present in this way. Remember that when eliciting the history, clues can be obtained from the patient regarding the diagnosis, e.g. mid-cycle pain in the female (Mittelschmertz), prodromal illness (mesenteric adenitis), weight loss and diarrhoea (possible Crohn's disease). A rectal examination is largely unhelpful, although many consultants will insist on one being performed, so be aware of your seniors' wishes! However, rectal examination should never be performed in children.

The basic principles of fluid resuscitation and analgesia apply here as for an acute abdomen, particularly in the extremes of age, where very young or the elderly can become toxic due to dehydration and sepsis rather dramatically. Unless you have made a definite clinical diagnosis of appendicitis or another cause of RIF pain has been found, such as a urinary tract infection (UTI), antibiotics should not be administered. Helpful blood tests include the leucocyte count and the CRP, but normal blood results do not rule out appendicitis, since the diagnosis is a clinical one. Similarly, the role of imaging is secondary. Plain radiographs should not be requested, and there is continued discussion as to the usefulness of abdominal ultrasound (US). In females with RIF pain, don't forget to check the result of a pregnancy test as such patients with a positive pregnancy test are assumed to have an ectopic pregnancy until proven otherwise. If other gynaecological causes are suspected, a pelvic and/or trans-vaginal US can be useful, and will always be required before you request a gynaecological review! Older patients with appendicitis are less common, and most will warrant a CT scan to rule out other pathology such as diverticulitis or sinister causes such as caecal carcinoma. This will need to be requested by a registrar or consultant.

Ultimately, if you strongly suspect appendicitis, then keep the patient nil by mouth, call your registrar and if appropriate within your capabilities, alert theatres and consent the patient. If you are in doubt, admit the patient for observation, since the clinical picture can change within hours. Beware the patient that has been sent home with unexplained RIF pain on more than one occasion; these patients are usually admitted for further investigations, but if deemed fit, should always be reviewed by someone senior to you prior to discharge from the emergency deparment. Finally, if your registrar agrees that the patient has appendicitis, try and perform the operation with them.

Herniae

Abdominal wall herniae that commonly present in the emergency department include inguinal, femoral, paraumbilical, incisional and ventral. Common to all of them is the risk of incarceration, intestinal obstruction and strangulation. Usually the diagnosis is made on clinical assessment alone, although abdominal radiographs are useful to rule out bowel obstruction. If the overlying skin is discoloured, or there is abnormal physiology, then strangulation must be considered, and these herniae, together with those associated with bowel obstruction usually require prompt surgical intervention, whilst painful incarcerated herniae can often be managed conservatively, so initial management is crucial.

If clinical assessment and radiography confirm obstruction, then call your registrar without delay. Ensure the patient has adequate IV access and is being rehydrated. Catheterise the patient and ask the nurses to record fluid balance. Arrange for an NG tube to be inserted to decompress the bowel. Keep the patient nil by mouth and mark the hernia site. Depending on the age and co-morbidities of the patient, you may need to alert the anaesthetist on call, since the patient may require optimisation pre- and post-surgically in a high dependency unit. Your registrar should review and consent the patient, since patients with obstructed herniae frequently require laparotomy and resection of small or large bowel, which is not appropriate for F2/CT consent.

Patients with painful herniae but without clinical or radiological signs of obstruction may be managed conservatively in the first instance. They also require fluid resuscitation and appropriate analgesia. In some cases, after the administration of strong analgesia, the hernia can be reduced, eliminating the need for emergency surgery. Providing it is reducible, and depending on local protocol, these patients can then either be discharged and brought back for elective surgery, or admitted and treated surgically on the first available appropriate list. Ensure you know what your hospital policy is.

Knowledge of basic inguinal and femoral anatomy is essential in case you end up being questioned by the consultant!

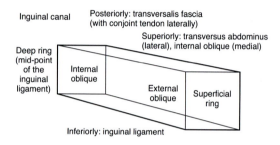

FIGURE 1.1 Inguinal anatomy.

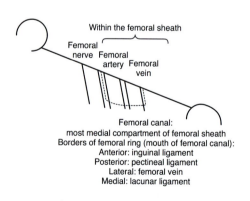

FIGURE 1.2 Femoral anatomy.

Gallstone disease

Most gallstones are asymptomatic, but when problems occur, patients present with a clinical spectrum ranging from biliary colic to pancreatitis (*see* 'Pancreatitis', pp. 12–14). The most likely presenting feature is epigastric or right upper quadrant (RUQ) pain together with bloating and post-prandial discomfort, although in the presence of cholecystitis, sepsis can be the main problem. Examination findings will include any or all of the following: tachycardia, fever, RUQ pain (including Murphy's sign positivity), RUQ mass, jaundice, peritonitis and shock.

The initial management will be as for all cases of acute abdomen, i.e. resuscitation and stabilisation together with analgesia. Investigations will include full blood count, urea and electrolytes, liver function tests, amylase, clotting screen, CRP and a group and save. Imaging is also indicated (see below). Simple biliary colic may not require admission; BSG guidelines state that wherever possible, patients presenting with biliary colic for the first time should be investigated with ultrasound, and if proven to have gallstones, should have a cholecystectomy (preferably laparoscopically) on that admission. However, in practice, service capacity varies from hospital to hospital, and most patients with simple biliary colic responding to paracetamol or oral opioid analgesia will be sent home for outpatient investigation and follow-up. You should check local policy in your hospital. The other conditions associated with gallstones should ideally be managed as below.

Cholecystitis

Patients presenting with biliary colic in the presence of sepsis can be assumed to have cholecystitis, and the diagnosis can be made on clinical grounds alone. Patients are usually admitted and commenced on IV antibiotics according to local guidelines, often Tazocin® or Timentin®. Fluid resuscitation is important and a strict fluid balance chart should be initiated. Simple erect chest radiography should rule out other causes of RUQ pain and fever, such as a perforated viscus or right lower lobe pneumonia. Although an abdominal radiograph is unhelpful in the diagnosis, occasionally gallstones may be seen. Urgent ultrasound should be arranged and the patient kept on clear fluids.

Empyema

Where the gall bladder is full of infected mucus or pus, the resultant distension can usually render the gall bladder palpable. Often empyema is associated with the elderly, and septic shock may be a presenting feature, which should be immediately addressed. Patients should be catheterised for accurate fluid assessment, IV antibiotics commenced and urgent ultrasound +/– guided drainage should be arranged. These patients need early review by your registrar.

Cholangitis

Cholangitis is a potentially life-threatening condition arising from sepsis involving the biliary tree, and is usually caused by an impacted stone or stones in the common bile duct. Needless to say, urgent resuscitation is crucial, and these patients need immediate review by your registrar, as a large proportion of patients will need further assessment by intensive care with a view to admission. Ensure the patient is catheterised and IV antibiotics commenced. Guidelines suggest that prompt intervention with ERCP should follow, but again due to service limitations, this is not always possible. Beware those patients with cholangitis who have an underlying malignancy rather than gallstones; your registrar will need to arrange further imaging in the form of CT or MRI as required.

Pancreatitis

Although everyone seems to remember scorpion bites as a cause of pancreatitis, the three commonest causes in the UK are gallstones, alcohol and drugs. Largely for historic reasons (previously, pancreatitis was frequently treated by debridement and necrosectomy), the condition is usually managed by surgeons. Unfortunately, pancreatitis is still a cause of death, predominantly amongst the elderly or the immunocompromised, and therefore the initial diagnosis needs no delay and management should be aggressive. Patients will frequently have a history of increased alcohol intake, often binge drinking immediately before an attack. However, previous heavy drinkers are often affected after only one or two drinks. The presence of jaundice is usually an indicator of gallstones, although of course severe liver disease secondary to alcohol can be a cause. The diagnosis is usually made by the presence of hyperamylasaemia, usually at least 2.5–3 times the upper limit of normal reference values. In chronic pancreatitis, however, the amylase is frequently normal. Some centres use pancreatic lipase, as it is far more specific, but use of this tool is not widespread. Other important blood tests to request are the usual full blood count (FBC), urea and electrolytes, LFTs, CRP and glucose. If you strongly suspect pancreatitis before the amylase levels are back, then it is a good idea to request a calcium level as well.

Since amylase levels can also be increased in other intra-abdominal catastrophes such as perforated viscus, an erect chest radiograph should be requested. Occasionally, if an abdominal X-ray is performed, a sentinel loop of small bowel or calcification of the pancreas may be visible. Once the diagnosis of pancreatitis has been confirmed, it is important to commence urgent fluid resuscitation and administer analgesia and anti-emetics. Concurrently, a prognostic scoring system should be used according to local protocol, such as Ranson, Glasgow or APACHE. Most hospitals have these to download from the intranet; make sure you know where to look! The scoring system will ensure that important investigations are not missed, such as arterial blood gas and specific blood tests such as calcium and LDH/AST. Guidelines suggest patients with an initial Ranson or Glasgow score of <3 can be safely managed on the ward with accurate fluid balance, oxygen and IV fluids. An NG tube is not mandatory, but may help nausea and vomiting. Similarly, catheterisation can be used judiciously. Where patients score ≥3, prompt registrar review is essential, since these patients should be managed in an HDU setting, or at the very least, require an ITU review. Such patients MUST have both an NG tube and a urinary catheter. The usefulness of antibiotics is not proven; antibiotics are only useful in the presence of pancreatic necrosis or concurrent cholangitis. Therefore, in patients scoring <3, antibiotics should not be prescribed, whilst in acute severe pancreatitis, antibiotics may be given but only after discussion with the microbiologist or where there is proven necrosis.

Further imaging will need to be arranged; ultrasound is usually required to look for gallstones and to investigate the calibre of the common bile duct. Where gallstones are the cause of pancreatitis, guidelines suggest either ERCP within 48 hours or cholecystectomy on that admission, depending on the presence or absence of biliary obstruction. Again, service provision will dictate whether this can be achieved. CT scanning is not useful in the first 3–5 days, since oedema will preclude useful characterisation of the pancreas. If patients do not settle within this time, then CT scanning will allow necrosis or pseudocyst formation to be diagnosed. Other serious complications include respiratory complications such as acute lung injury/ARDS, and if patients continue to be unwell with pancreatitis, obtaining a PaO_2 is important to exclude impending respiratory failure.

Diverticulitis

Patients with acute diverticulitis are commonly admitted on the surgical take. Remember the spectrum of disease can vary – from localised abdominal tenderness to the patient with signs and symptoms of peritonitis. Beware of the elderly or immunocompromised patient who may not present with all the signs of intra-abdominal sepsis.

The Hinchey classification helps to classify the stages of disease severity (radiologically or intraoperatively):

- ➲ **Stage 1**: Diverticulitis with localised abscess (pericolic or mesenteric).
- ➲ **Stage 2**: Diverticulitis with walled off pelvic abscess.
- ➲ **Stage 3**: Diverticulitis with generalised purulent peritonitis.
- ➲ **Stage 4**: Diverticulitis with generalised faecal peritonitis.

If the patient is unwell, inform your registrar and then continue to reassess and resuscitate the patient. As for all acute surgical admissions, take a thorough but focused history – remembering to ask about change in bowel habit, rectal bleeding and urinary symptoms (the sigmoid diverticulitis may be irritating the bladder or they may have pneumaturia, which would indicate a colovesical fistula). Ask about previous investigations, as many will be known to have diverticulosis. A rectal examination should be performed. Initial investigations should be an FBC, U&E, CRP, blood cultures if pyrexial and a urinalysis. A plain AXR is unlikely to show anything specific but an erect CXR should be requested, to exclude a perforation. Intravenous fluids and antibiotics should be prescribed, along with regular analgesia. Consider catheterisation if the patient is septic and accurate fluid balance is required. Some patients may need an urgent laparotomy (a Hartmann's procedure will usually be performed) and transfer to ITU. Your registrar should consent the patient, but you can check a group and save and inform theatres, the anaesthetist and the patient's relatives.

Patients with localised diverticulitis and mild abdominal tenderness may settle with a short course of intravenous antibiotics and be discharged with an oral course and dietary information. Further investigations are usually needed but seem to vary according to consultant, so ask before requesting them! An outpatient flexible sigmoidoscopy (at least 6 weeks after discharge, to allow the inflammation to settle) is often suitable. Patients with more severe disease, will usually need a CT scan to exclude complications of diverticulitis (abscess, fistula, localised perforation). If the patient is stable, this may not need to be performed out of hours, so discuss with your registrar. Remember an INR will be needed if radiological drainage is performed.

Obstruction

Patients presenting with 'abdominal pain and vomiting – query obstruction' will frequently be referred to the surgical team. A targeted history and thorough abdominal examination will help you decide if they do indeed have bowel obstruction, the site and the likely cause. Think about other causes of pain and vomiting, such as gastroenteritis or exacerbation of IBD, and prepare to refer to the medical team if you think this is the cause.

Common surgical causes are:

- ⤷ underlying malignancy – ask about change in bowel habit, PR bleeding, weight loss and family history of bowel cancer
- ⤷ adhesions from previous abdominal operations – they may not always remember, so inspect the abdomen carefully (appendicectomies were not always performed laparoscopically or by a Lanz incision!)
- ⤷ hernia (umbilical, inguinal, femoral, incisional) – beware as the elderly unwell patient may not be able to tell you about their groin lump, so careful examination is needed
- ⤷ volvulus (most commonly sigmoid) – may have had previous episodes (check previous imaging if poor historian), ask about bowel habit and note their medications.

On examination, the patient may be very dehydrated, tachycardic and hypotensive. Simultaneous resuscitation and assessment may be needed and you must repeatedly review them to ensure they are responding to the fluids and analgesia you have prescribed. Look for abdominal distension and scars, percuss to see if they are tympanic, note the areas of tenderness or presence of a mass. Be sure to check the hernial orifices, as it will be very embarrassing to miss an obvious groin swelling! Listen for bowel sounds and perform a rectal examination. Check FBC, U&E, glucose and an ABG – they may be hypokalaemic, so correct electrolytes promptly. Order an erect CXR and AXR. Insert a catheter for strict fluid balance and an NG tube and ask for hourly urine output. An ECG should be requested, oxygen given as needed and adequate analgesia and antiemetics should be prescribed. Don't use metoclopramide as this is a prokinetic, which will make the problem worse. If they have an acute kidney injury, remember to omit their nephrotoxic drugs. The U&E and ABG may need to be repeated later to check they are improving.

Remember to call your registrar early if the patient is unwell and ITU/outreach should be informed early on. Many patients will need a period of fluid resuscitation (drip and suck) but some will need an urgent CT scan and others will require prompt surgery.

If the AXR shows a sigmoid volvulus, this will need decompression – this can usually be achieved on the ward, with a rigid sigmoidoscope and insertion of flatus tube. You will need to learn how to do this. Be warned – tie your hair back, wear a large apron, roll your sleeves up and watch your shoes! If you are unable to decompress with a rigid sigmoidoscopy, discuss with your senior as this patient may well need a flexible sigmoidoscopy to reach the point of volvulus.

Acute mesenteric ischaemia

Although this is not a common surgical admission, you should be aware that it has a high mortality rate and so a rapid diagnosis is important. It is caused by a sudden reduction of blood flow to a large part of the bowel, leading to irreversible full thickness bowel ischaemia. Therefore, the patient may present with sudden onset, generalised and severe abdominal pain.

It may be caused by the following:

- ⮑ mesenteric artery embolism
- ⮑ mesenteric artery thrombosis
- ⮑ mesenteric venous thrombosis
- ⮑ non-occlusive arterial hypotension – most commonly mesenteric vasoconstriction secondary to reduced cardiac output (MI).

> **Remember to ask about risk factors:**
> - ⮑ atherosclerosis
> - ⮑ increasing age
> - ⮑ cardiac arrythmias (AF)/recent MI/valve disease
> - ⮑ smoking
> - ⮑ diabetes.

On examination, the abdomen may be soft with only mild widespread tenderness. Note the pain is often out of proportion to the examination findings. Request an FBC (WCC may be raised), U&E, INR, G&S and perform an ABG (usually shows a severe metabolic acidosis with a high lactate). Administer oxygen and IV fluids and ask for an ECG. The patient may be fit for urgent surgery, so alert your senior early. A CT scan may not be helpful as it is not very sensitive for detecting bowel wall ischaemia. If the patient is not fit for surgical intervention, discussions with the patient and family will be needed and you must ensure the patient is kept comfortable with regular strong analgesia.

Rectal bleeding

There are many causes of rectal bleeding and a careful history will hopefully help you to identify the most likely cause.

When you are clerking the patient, be sure to ask the following:

- ➲ colour of the blood – bright red/dark red/clots? Be sure it is not melaena (as this is usually admitted under the medics!). Patients find it hard to quantify the amount (and will often overestimate) but measuring it in 'teaspoons or cupfuls' sometimes helps
- ➲ painful/painless – an anal fissure is exquisitely painful (like passing 'broken glass') whereas haemorrhoidal bleeding is usually painless
- ➲ occurrence – with every bowel motion/mixed in or separate from the stool
- ➲ stool frequency and vomiting – could be due to gastroenteritis
- ➲ associated abdominal pain (may be diverticulitis)
- ➲ weight loss/recent change in bowel habit (may indicate underlying malignancy)
- ➲ co-morbidities – AF, metallic heart valves, recent MI – as this will be relevant if anticoagulant/antiplatelet reversal is needed
- ➲ medications – e.g. warfarin/aspirin/clopidogrel.

On examinaton, take a careful note of the baseline observations and watch for changes. Before performing the rectal examination, ensure the patient is lying in the correct position and there is good light – you do not want to miss obvious pathology that will easily be seen on a daylight ward round. Look for skin tags/prolapsed haemorrhoids/blood and inspect carefully for an anal fissure. On digital examination, feel for stool consistency/any masses and the presence of blood. Request an FBC, INR and a G&S/cross-match if large volume rectal bleeding. Consider if an AXR is really indicated but always ask for a stool chart to be kept.

If the patient has had significant rectal bleeding or is haemodynamically unstable, wide-bore IV access should be obtained and prompt resuscitation commenced. They may require a blood transfusion. A high INR with ongoing bleeding will require treatment and you should speak to the Haematologist on call for advice. Most patients will settle with conservative management and will need a flexible sigmoidoscopy/colonoscopy when the bleeding has ceased. If they remain unstable, a CT angiogram may be helpful. Equally, you need to consider whether this may be a high-volume upper gastrointestinal bleed, which will require OGD.

At the other end of the spectrum, patients with prolapsed haemorrhoids may be treated with covered icepacks, simple analgesia, laxatives and not require admission. Similarly, patients with anal fissures may also be discharged with treatment (diltiazem/GTN ointment and laxatives) and surgical follow-up.

Rectal prolapse

Common risk factors:
- ➲ constipation
- ➲ chronic cough
- ➲ pelvic floor dysfunction (multiple pregnancies)
- ➲ psychiatric disease.

Rectal prolapse is protrusion of the rectal mucosa or entire rectal wall through the anus. It frequently occurs on straining or even standing and most commonly affects elderly ladies. Many of them will have had it for years without seeking medical attention. Often you will only be called when it is painful and irreducible. It may look ulcerated or slightly dusky and be bleeding. The most important thing you can do is reduce it quickly. This will require good analgesia (Oramorph or Entonox) as the patient needs to be relaxed. They will need to be lying on their side comfortably as they will be there for a while.

There are many techniques and tactics to aid reduction, but essentially you need to try and reduce the amount of oedema present in the bowel wall. Constant pressure (not the squeeze and peek technique) will help. You may need an osmotic agent, like table sugar (yes, really!), to draw the oedema out of the bowel wall.

If you are unable to reduce the prolapse, call your registrar. It is highly likely that they will be able to reduce it. After reduction, make sure you prescribe laxatives to minimise straining. You will want to think about longer-term management, particularly if this is a recurrent event. Surgical intervention is normally done electively and patients will need an anaesthetic assessment as they often have many co-morbidities.

Abscesses

Patients with perianal and pilonidal abscesses are commonly referred to the surgical take but those with infected sebaceous cysts (back/shoulder) will also be seen. Women with breast abscesses are less frequently admitted as they can often be booked directly into the breast clinic for an ultrasound scan (USS) +/– aspiration.

We are always taught the adage, 'never let the sun set on undrained pus', but nowadays a lot of hospitals have an abscess pathway where the patient goes home, returns the next day and is the first case on the emergency list. Make sure you know your hospital policy. The pathway may not be appropriate if they are elderly/frail or systemically unwell/pyrexial.

Treatment of an abscess is incision and drainage under general anaesthetic. Bear this in mind when you are clerking the patient and request the appropriate investigations (ECG, bloods) to ensure theatre is not delayed.

Be careful to note the following:

- diabetes – will they need a sliding scale? How is their blood sugar control, as this may contribute to poor wound healing
- immunocompromise – this will impact on wound healing, length of stay
- previous abscesses
- medications – e.g. warfarin – their INR must be checked pre-operatively
- intravenous drug users – these patients commonly have groin abscesses and a USS must always be ordered to ensure there is not a false aneurysm.

The abscess should be marked (as appropriate) and the patient consented if you are able. For those with perianal abscesses, they may also need a rigid sigmoidoscopy, insertion of seton or laying open of fistula-in-ano, so make sure this is included on the consent form – if you are unable to consent for this, your registrar will need to. Patients with a pilonidal abscess may require further (elective) surgery once the abscess has been drained and healed. If possible go to theatre and perform the incision and drainage.

Wound infection

Most wound infections are not seen by the surgical team as they are managed in the community by the GP. Risk factors for patients developing wound problems include raised BMI, diabetes, smoking and immunocompromise. Stoma closures and umbilical wounds are more likely to get infected. Make sure you take a targeted history – what operation did the patient have and when was it?

Make sure the patient isn't septic by checking the temperature and observations. Examine the wound and ensure there is no fluctuance as there may be a collection that needs incision and drainage or a haematoma that needs evacuating. This may need to be performed under general anaesthetic, so prepare the patient in the usual fashion for theatre. If the patient is systemically well and the wound has surrounding erythema only, a course of oral antibiotics may suffice. Blood tests may not always be needed, but a wound swab is helpful.

There are a couple of things to watch out for. A small bowel fistula may present as ongoing discharge from a wound that is failing to heal. In hernia repairs where a mesh (biological or synthetic) has been used, you may need to treat more aggressively, perhaps with IV antibiotics, as mesh infections can be disastrous.

Chapter 2

VASCULAR SURGERY

Matthew Stephenson

The acutely ischaemic limb

Ischaemic limbs are the bread and butter of vascular surgery, although the vast majority in clinical practice are chronically ischaemic. For those clinicians without much vascular experience the ischaemic limb is perhaps one of the most misunderstood emergencies. The classic six Ps presentation (see below) is relatively uncommon and in fact most legs presenting acutely have acute-on-chronic ischaemia. Nevertheless, let's start with the most obvious, pressing emergency: acute ischaemia.

Acute leg ischaemia

Presentation

History:

- ➲ sudden onset of severe foot pain, which always affects at least the most distal part of the leg
- ➲ the leg may feel numb, parasthetic or weak.

Examination:

- ➲ painful (or more accurately tender)
- ➲ pale
- ➲ pulseless
- ➲ parasthetic (or more accurately, reduced sensation)
- ➲ perishingly cold
- ➲ paralysed.

Aetiology

Thrombotic, e.g.:

- ➲ thrombosis on a pre-existing arterial atherosclerotic lesion
- ➲ thrombotic occlusion of a popliteal aneurysm.

Embolic, e.g.:

⮑ usually cardiac but can be from the aorta.

Pain and pulselessness are the most consistent features. As ischaemia progresses, the patient will then develop ischaemia of the sensory and motor nerves, which accounts for the later reduced sensation and paralysis. An insensate paralysed leg is very ischaemic indeed and almost certainly beyond salvage. Furthermore, tender muscle compartments are a sign of severe muscle ischaemia and risk of compartment syndrome (make sure you compress the calf and the anterior compartment for tenderness). The initial pallor gives way after time to a dusky appearance as cutaneous vasodilatation occurs. A mottled appearance develops, which at first blanches on pressure. When the mottling no longer blanches, this indicates the capillaries have burst and the leg is probably unsalvageable. Fortunately, there is a system to help you establish the severity of the ischaemic limb – to help you prioritise at 3am, see the table of clinical categories of acute limb ischaemia below.

Table I. Clinical categories of acute limb ischaemia

Category	Description/prognosis	Findings		Doppler signals	
		Sensory loss	Muscle weakness	Arterial	Venous
I. Viable	Not immediately threatened	None	None	Audible	Audible
II. Threatened					
a. Marginally	Salvageable if promptly treated	Minimal (toes) or none	None	Inaudible	Audible
b. Immediately	Salvageable with immediate revascularization	More than toes, associated with rest pain	Mild, moderate	Inaudible	Audible
III. Irreversible	Major tissue loss or permanent nerve damage inevitables	Profound, anesthetic	Profound, paralysis (rigor)	Inaudible	Inaudible

(Reprinted with permission from Rutherford RB, Baker JD, Ernst C, *et al.* Recommended standards for reports dealing with lower extremity ischemia: revised version. *J Vasc Surg.* 2007; **26**(3): 517–38. Copyright Elsevier 2007.)

What to do

Initial steps

- ⊃ You must thoroughly examine the patient to confirm the diagnosis and establish the severity, and this *must* include examination of the pulses with a Doppler probe. Even if you can't feel the pulses, the presence of a normal triphasic Doppler signal in the foot reassures you that the foot is not ischaemic.
- ⊃ You must discuss the case with a vascular surgeon. The things most junior doctors forget to check before picking up the phone are: sensory loss, muscle weakness and compartment tenderness.
- ⊃ Proceed with investigations.

Investigations: this is a complex issue. Sometimes, when the diagnosis is barn door obvious, no investigations are necessary and the patient should proceed straight to theatre. When it's unclear, the patient should have imaging in some form but this depends hugely on local policy and availability. The options are:

- ⊃ duplex ultrasound
- ⊃ CT angiogram
- ⊃ MR angiogram
- ⊃ digital subtraction angiogram.

The latter option has the benefit of also being able to proceed with therapeutic angioplasty or thrombolysis if required but this should all be discussed with a vascular surgeon +/– interventional radiologist.

Also, the non-specific tests:

- ⊃ lab: full blood count, U&E, clotting, group and save
- ⊃ other: ECG, chest X-ray.

Treatment

- ⊃ IV fluid resuscitation.
- ⊃ IV heparin – follow your local protocol but usually consists of 5000 units stat followed by an infusion. Draw up 20 000 units (in 20 mL) and give 1 mL/hr, i.e. 1000 units heparin per hour. This keeps the microcirculation open and prevents clot propagation. Remember this would need to be stopped 90 minutes before any neuroaxial anaesthetic block to keep the anaesthetist happy. However, many vascular surgeons will be happy to operate whilst the patient is heparinised – this is a decision for them to make.
- ⊃ Analgesia.
- ⊃ 24% O_2.
- ⊃ Treat concomitant medical conditions, i.e. cardiac failure.

The definitive treatment depends on the presentation and results of investigations and is the subject of a whole other book but broadly can be:

- ⊃ Open:
  - embolectomy (for embolic causes)
  - arterial bypass (broadly speaking, for thrombotic/ occlusive causes)
  - primary amputation (for unsalvageable limbs).

OR

- ⊃ Endovascular:
  - thrombolysis
  - angioplasty.
- ⊃ Conservative:
  - palliative care, where this is part of an end-of-life process.

Acute-on-chronic leg ischaemia

Far more common is the chronically ischaemic leg with an acute deterioration. These patients usually have a claudication history and also diminished contralateral pulses. They rarely present with the six Ps as they have had time to build up a collateral circulation. They more commonly present with increasing pain or tissue loss (gangrene, ulceration). These present less of a hyperacute emergency. The investigative and treatment pathway as described above should be followed. However, time is more on your side and investigations and treatment are usually achieved over 24–48 hours rather than a few hours. Nevertheless, unless you're very comfortable with the situation at 03:00 it is best to take the advice of the vascular surgeon on call.

Abdominal aortic aneurysms

This is one of the true emergencies facing the surgeon and can be extremely daunting for the new surgical SHO in the middle of the night. Abdominal aortic aneurysms (AAAs) must be diagnosed and treated promptly if the patient is to have any chance of survival. Fortunately, the presentation is usually quite profound and obvious although many other general surgical emergencies can mimic it in part. The classic presentation is described below, but with an increasingly obese population, for instance, a pulsatile mass may be impossible to feel, or sometimes the pain can be solely in the back.

Presentation

History

⮕ Sudden onset severe abdominal pain radiating through to the back.

⮕ Collapse, with or without loss of consciousness.

Examination

⮕ Shock.

⮕ A tender pulsatile abdominal mass.

What to do

Initial steps

⮕ Summon senior help immediately if you've diagnosed an AAA – this will usually be in the form of the vascular registrar on call, or the general surgical registrar if you don't have vascular on-site.

⮕ Obtain large-bore IV access × 2, *but*:
  ● don't give any IV fluids or blood yet! If a patient has survived an initial aneurysm rupture it is because the

retroperitoneum has tamponaded the bleed temporarily – if you give injudicious IV fluids the patient may suddenly exsanguinate. As long as the patient is conscious, even a systolic blood pressure of 70 will have to do for now.

- ➲ Alert the anaesthetic team.
- ➲ Proceed with investigations as necessary.

Specific investigations

These depend on the certainty of your diagnosis and the availability of imaging. There are two modalities to image the aorta in this emergency circumstance.

1 Duplex – very quick, can be performed in resus without having to move the patient. This procedure will tell you if there is an AAA but won't necessarily tell you if it's leaking. If the aorta is 2.5 cm, it isn't a leaking AAA. If the aorta is 6 cm, it's an AAA but you can't be sure if it's leaking.

2 CT aortogram – extremely accurate at assessing the aorta and detecting a leak. It also allows you to plan whether the AAA would be suitable for emergency endovascular aneurysm repair (EVAR) (if available at your hospital). However, the CT scanner isn't nicknamed the 'doughnut of death' for nothing – unstable patients have a habit of arresting in CT.

A patient with a known 8 cm AAA, awaiting elective repair with the classic presentation described above has an AAA – no debate required. He should proceed immediately to theatre for repair. The only reason he might have a CTA is if he is stable and there is an option to do emergency EVAR. At the other extreme, a patient with no known AAA history with abdominal and back pain and history of collapse but is now cardiovascularly stable should have a CT scan to confirm the diagnosis. In the middle is a grey area and decisions are taken on a case-by-case basis in discussion with the vascular team.

General investigations
- ⊃ Lab: full blood count, U&E, clotting, group and save with 6-unit cross-match.
- ⊃ Other: ECG, arterial blood gas, chest X-ray (mobile).

Next steps:

If you have a confirmed diagnosis of a ruptured AAA, here is a checklist of things you must make sure are done *right now* – you have very little time and must be organised:
- ⊃ vascular surgeons aware and en route
- ⊃ the anaesthetic registrar on call is aware and en route
- ⊃ theatres are aware – this is a CEPOD category 1 emergency!
- ⊃ the blood bank is aware (you will need a massive transfusion pack ready – they will prepare platelets, blood and FFP)
- ⊃ ITU is aware (the patient will need to go there afterwards)
- ⊃ all venous bloods are sent off (as above)
- ⊃ the cell saver (for autotransfusion) is available in theatre and someone knows how to use it.

Treatment

The only treatment for a ruptured AAA is surgical repair, either with traditional open repair via a laparotomy or EVAR. Leave the specifics of this, for now, to the vascular team and focus on confirming the diagnosis and ensuring the above checklist is complete. Your role is often as a coordinator to ensure that the patient progresses smoothly to theatre – it may seem menial but it saves lives. In case you're on your own in theatre and the vascular surgeon hasn't arrived yet, make sure the following happen whilst you're waiting:

- ➲ insert a urinary catheter and attach to a urometer
- ➲ shave the patient from nipples to knees
- ➲ make sure the results of the CT (if performed) are available on the computer
- ➲ check the family know what's happening and try to get as much collateral history as possible
- ➲ make sure that the cell saver is available
- ➲ confirm with the blood bank that they have a massive transfusion pack ready
- ➲ help the anaesthetist if needed with any lines/further blood samples
- ➲ if you're confident and have done prepping and draping before, and the surgeon still hasn't arrived, prep the skin from nipples to knees, place a sterile towel over the genitals and drape the whole prepped area so that from xiphisternum to knee level is exposed. The patient will still be awake as you do this because the anaesthetist will not induce anaesthesia until knife is about to be applied to skin as the induction agent compounds the hypotension resulting sometimes in a very rapid need for a clamp on the aorta.

Acute aortic dissection

When there is a breach in the aortic endothelium, blood can track into the arterial media producing a false track – a 'dissection'. This can result in a number of clinical sequelae depending on what happens next as this track can either extend:

- ➲ out of the aorta and leak freely, i.e. a rapidly fatal rupture
- ➲ in an antegrade direction separating the true lumen from the various arterial ostia causing organ ischaemia
- ➲ in a retrograde direction causing a rapidly fatal pericardial tamponade, aortic valve incompetence or coronary ischaemia
- ➲ back into the true lumen (if the patient is lucky).

Remember also that aortic dissection can be seen in the chronic setting (defined as present for >2 weeks), where the initial episode may even have gone unnoticed and the dissection flap has stabilised. These are a slightly different entity.

Presentation

History

- ➲ Severe sharp/tearing chest pain radiating through to the back.
- ➲ Background of hypertension.

Examination

- ➲ Stroke (occlusion of the carotid arteries).
- ➲ Arm ischaemia (occlusion of the brachiocephalic or sub-clavian arteries).
- ➲ Paralysis (occlusion of the spinal arteries).

- Renal failure (occlusion of the renal arteries).
- Ischaemic gut (occlusion of the visceral arteries).
- Ischaemic leg (occlusion of the iliac or femoral arteries).
- Collapse/hypotension (rupture or pericardial tamponade).

What to do

It is generally difficult to diagnose a thoracic aortic dissection without investigations – it could be a myocardial infarction or pulmonary embolus for example. Therefore, the A&E department will almost always have done the preliminary cardiac work first, specifically an ECG and troponin. If these are negative, the patient needs a CT aortogram, usually A&E organise this and you are referred a patient with a radiologically proven thoracic dissection.

The key thing to check on the CTA (or ask the radiologist) is:

- Is this a Stanford type A dissection? – involves (at least) the ascending aorta. The management has suddenly become very straightforward for you; the patient needs urgent cardiothoracic referral. These dissections always need surgical repair to replace the root of the aorta. This is a true emergency with 1% mortality per hour.
- Is this a Stanford type B dissection? – does not involve the aortic root. The next thing you need to establish is: are there any of the complications listed above in the presentation section? If so, this is a complicated Type B dissection and may need surgery. If there is none of the above present, this patient will not need surgery (for now at least) and should be managed by the medics/cardiologists to obtain scrupulous blood pressure control (in order to reduce the risk of dissection extension). In any event, discuss with a vascular surgeon.

Treatment

Type A: urgent surgical repair.

Type B – uncomplicated: as above, meticulous blood pressure control (often requires intravenous antihypertensive infusions).

Type B – complicated: as above, likely to need surgery. This involves two aspects:

- ➲ closure of the dissection. Now almost always by an endovascular stent passed transfemorally, which presses the dissecting flap back against the wall and redirects the blood through the true lumen. Open repair is now rare, as very high mortality
- ➲ revascularisation of ischaemic organs. Specifics depend on the organ affected but may include, for example, a femoro-femoral bypass for an occluded iliac artery.

Leg ulcers

An ulcer is a breach in an epithelial surface, in this case, the skin of the leg or foot. It is not uncommon for A&E, or for GPs, to refer leg ulcers to the surgeon on call, usually because they don't know what to do with them, and sometimes the cause is vascular (although the treatment is actually uncommonly surgical). The aetiology for leg ulcers is important to remember when managing them. The following mnemonic may help:

Venous Superficial venous incompetence (varicose veins).
Deep venous incompetence (i.e. post-DVT). For the purposes of this mnemonic, as they all involve high pressure, this also includes:
- dependency oedema
- lymphoedema.

Arterial Macrovascular (atherosclerosis).
Microvascular (small vessel disease as seen in diabetes mellitus, connective tissue diseases, etc.).

Trauma To neuropathic skin (often diabetic neuropathy).
To normally innervated skin (for instance decubitus ulcers).

Infective Infection is a common complication of pre-existent ulcers but very rarely there may be an exotic tropical cause, i.e. cutaneous leishmaniasis.

Neoplastic Arising de novo (i.e. ulcerating basal cell carcinoma).
Arising from chronic ulceration (Marjolin's ulcer).

Of course, sometimes it is caused by a combination of these. To diagnose the cause of the ulcer, therefore, you need to go through this list eliminating aetiologies and much can be done on the history and examination.

Presentation

History

- ⮕ Any history of varicose veins? Ever had surgery for varicose veins? Ever had a DVT?
- ⮕ Have they experienced claudication or ischaemic rest pain? What are their risk factors for atherosclerosis?
- ⮕ Do they have a history of diabetes mellitus? For how long? Do they have any diagnosis of connective tissue disease? Any joint pains? Are they on steroids?
- ⮕ Have they noticed any change in their sensation (they often don't) or parasthaesia?
- ⮕ Do they remember any trauma?
- ⮕ Have they been immobile (in the case of ulcers over pressure points or dependency oedema)?
- ⮕ Have they had any recent travel abroad?
- ⮕ How did the ulcer start (e.g. from a raised lesion)? Where relevant, have they noticed a growth on the ulcer?

Examination

- ⮕ Check for varicose veins and listen with a Doppler probe at the saphenofemoral and saphenopopliteal junctions for incompetence.
- ⮕ Look for signs of chronic venous insufficiency:
  - haemosiderin deposition (brown pigmentation)
  - lipodermatosclerosis
  - venous eczema
  - oedema.

- Examine the arterial system (if they have a palpable foot pulse for example, the ulcer is not caused by macrovascular disease) including the ankle brachial pressure index.
- Examine sensation in the leg.
- Are there any suspicious raised lesions?
- Observe the characteristics of the ulcer (see below).

By far the commonest leg ulcers are either due to deep venous incompetence (usually post-DVT), dependency oedema or less commonly, arterial. The first two tend to look similar – they result from inadequate return of fluid from the leg either because the deep veins are incompetent or in dependency oedema there is inadequate muscle pump action to return blood in the veins or lymphatics. The leg is usually swollen and the ulcer is usually around the ankle, most commonly above the medial malleolus (the 'gaiter' area). It is shallow, with sloping edges and the base is usually a slough-covered granulation layer. They tend to be very painful.

In arterial ulceration, the foot must be critically ischaemic (usually chronically). The ulcer is always at the most distal point (where arterial blood has furthest to reach) or at pressure points (where the circulatory pressure must overcome extrinsic pressure). It is inconceivable that you could have arterial ulceration proximally in the leg but have a well-perfused foot distally (except at pressure points). The ulcer usually has a more 'punched out' appearance, i.e. the edges do not slope, they are perpendicular to the skin and base.

What to do

Investigations

Depending on the history and examination but may include:

- ⮕ FBC and inflammatory markers if concerned about infection
- ⮕ arterial or venous duplex if concerned about arterial or venous cause
- ⮕ suspicious lesions should be biopsied (although not usually in A&E, they should be referred, for instance, to a dermatologist).

Treatment

For arterial causes, i.e. an ischaemic leg – the management is of the ischaemic leg rather than the ulcer. The ulcer will heal when the foot regains its blood supply. In chronic cases the patient may be dischargeable back to an urgent vascular clinic or in more acute cases with recently ischaemic legs and progressive tissue loss, they should be admitted for inpatient assessment for revascularisation. This should be decided by a vascular surgeon.

For deep venous causes, lymphoedema or dependency oedema, the treatment is leg elevation and compression. This counteracts the high venous, lymphatic and tissue pressures. Often high-grade compression is required in the form of four-layer bandaging (which needs to be applied by someone expert in the procedure). Once the ulcer is healed, the patient should usually continue with Class II stockings indefinitely. Always examine the arterial system carefully before applying compression. There is no surgical cure for these problems.

For superficial venous incompetence (varicose veins), the patient should have leg elevation and compression just like above until the ulcer is healed. The varicose veins should then be surgically or endovascularly ablated.

Neuropathic ulceration needs careful attention to neuropathic areas with patient education and usually referral to a diabetic foot clinic. Superadded infection on top of ulcers usually requires antibiotics, in severe cases, as an inpatient. Malignant ulcers require wide local excision if suitable – rarely an amputation is required.

It gets more complicated when there is a mixture of causes, for instance a common one is a mixed arterial and venous ulcer. In this case you can't apply compression to the leg, as it will render it more ischaemic. The leg must be revascularised first, and then leg elevation or (mild-moderate) compression applied. This is why it is crucial to know the ABPIs before applying compression.

Usually the only ulcer presentation that may require emergency surgical admission is the one in the context of a severely ischaemic limb. The others can usually be managed in primary care or in follow-up with the relevant specialty in clinic. Infected venous or dependency ulcers sometimes require admission for antibiotics but more appropriately under the medics as these are essentially medically treated infections rather than anything stemming from a surgical target.

Chapter 3

UROLOGY

Elizabeth Bright and
Helen Teixeira

Acute urinary retention

Retention is fairly common. No registrar wants to be woken in the middle of the night to catheterise a patient, so it's important that you know how to deal with it.

This is not the time to practice your history and examination skills: imagine answering questions about your previous occupations whilst having over a litre of fluid in your bladder.

> **Bladder scanners are very easy to use**
> There are a variety of scanners on the wards, but they are easy to use and usually only have one button to negotiate. Place some jelly on the skin over the suprapubic area and point the scanner towards the bladder. Press the button and it will give you a reading in mL. Most scanners direct you to move up, down, left, right, etc. to ensure you have centralised the bladder and therefore get an accurate reading.

The following steps should see you through.

1 Quickly establish the diagnosis.
   ● How long since they last passed urine?
   ● Can you palpate a bladder (if not, a bladder scanner, if you can find one, may be useful).
2 Get a catheter in.
   ● The grumpiest patients will be singing your praises if you get that catheter in and relieve the pressure.
   ● Bigger is better, don't be tempted by the size 12 just because they have a big prostate.
3 Always record the residual volume and check the renal function.

- It's important to know how much urine was in the bladder.
- Monitor for diuresis. More than 200 mL an hour will require fluid replacement.
- Always dip the urine, as it will help you establish a cause (but remember there will always be blood due to catheter trauma).

4 Get the history.
- You can now take as long as you like to take the history and examine thoroughly.
- Don't forget to ask the important questions about the cause.

5 To go home or not to go home.
- Every hospital will have a different policy and it's important to know yours.
- Some departments will have a trial without catheter (TWOC) clinic, others will require liaising with district nurses.
- As a general rule of thumb any patient with evidence of diuresis or impaired renal function should stay for IV fluids.

Causes of retention

Urinary tract infection

The presence of nitrites in the urine dip is an indication of infection. Check your local guidelines for appropriate antibiotics.

Constipation

Constipation is a common cause of urinary retention in the elderly. This may require an enema, but beware of the mobility of your patient and their location. It's best to wait until they're on the ward and have easy access to a commode.

Prostatic hypertrophy

A long history of urinary tract symptoms such as hesitancy, poor stream and nocturia may indicate prostatic hypertrophy. You can consider starting an alpha-blocker such as tamsulosin; just make sure the GP is informed. If the patient fails their TWOC in the community despite an alpha blocker, they will require a urology outpatient appointment.

Prostatitis

These patients will present in severe pain often with signs of infection and sepsis. The prostate will be excruciatingly tender and prostatic massage may produce pus from the urethra (although I wouldn't advise this due to pain). Prescribe a course of antibiotics either orally or intravenous depending on how unwell the patient is. These patients may require suprapubic rather than urethral catheterisation.

Post-operative

These patients often have a pre-existing history of LUTS and will either have gone into retention post procedure or have failed a TWOC. They require re-catheterisation and another TWOC at a later date, preferably post-discharge when they are mobile and back to normal activities of daily living.

Neurological

When you've excluded other causes this is an important one to consider. Retention may occur in a patient with a known neurological diagnosis such as Parkinson's disease. However, in an otherwise fit and well patient, a new episode of acute retention, especially in women, should have you asking a few extra questions. Always do a neurological examination if there is any concern.

Alcohol

Common in middle-aged men who have had one too many drinks the night before! This causes over-distension of the bladder and therefore retention. Most will pass a TWOC 24–48 hours after catheterisation.

Alternatives to urethral catheterisation

If you are unable to insert a urethral catheter, don't panic, there are other tricks in the book. Never leave a patient overnight to be catheterised by the day team: they will be in a significant amount of pain.

Suprapubic catheters

If you have been taught how to insert a suprapubic catheter and you are confident that you can site one in this case, then do so. If you are not happy to perform suprapubic catheterisation, then there are other options.

Bladder aspiration

Insert a green needle attached to a syringe 2 cm above the pubic symphysis. Aspirate as you insert and once you are inside the bladder you will start to aspirate urine. Aspirate as much urine as possible and document the volume. You will not be able to completely empty the bladder, but it will make the patient more comfortable and give you time overnight before their bladder fills to capacity again. Definitive catheterisation can then be organised by the urology team in the morning.

Feeding tube

If the patient has a more complex surgical history, and you are concerned about damaging bowel with aspiration, this is a good alternative. A feeding NG tube can be inserted urethrally to drain the bladder. This can be taped to the patient to remain in overnight or removed after the bladder is emptied. Once again, by draining the bladder you have bought time overnight for definitive management in the morning.

Haematuria

Macroscopic haematuria, like retention, can be dealt with easily if you've got the know-how. As with retention, you want to deal with the immediate problem. Is there just haematuria or are they in clot retention? If in retention, catheterise!

The most time-consuming part of this will be gathering all of the kit together. Many of these items will be found in the urology ward or A&E.

Catheterisation

> **Kit you will need:**
> - three-way catheter
> - 50 mL bladder syringe
> - large catheter drainage bag
> - sterile water and syringe for the balloon (three-way catheters don't always come with a prefilled syringe)
> - spigot
> - sterile jug
> - bottle of sterile water
> - irrigation fluid plus giving set
> - bedpan/bowl (to drain any blood)
> - inco pads for the mess you're about to make.

Three-way catheters are designed with three ports:
- one for the balloon
- one for drainage
- one for irrigation.

They are generally larger than a normal catheter. This is for a good reason; you want to be able to drain large volumes of fluid and blood clots. Preferably put in a 22 or 24 French.

A three-way catheter balloon can be filled with 20–30 mL. It's important to document this so that the person removing the catheter removes all of the fluid from the balloon.

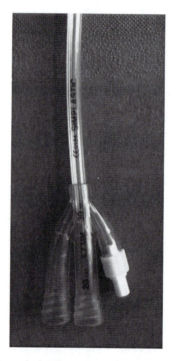

FIGURE 3.1 The end of a three-way catheter, with one port for drainage, one for the catheter balloon and the additional port for connection to irrigation fluid.

> **Bladder washout**
> - Always via the drainage port *not* via the irrigation port (spigot this or you will get wet).
> - Flush 50 mL into the bladder and aim to aspirate 50 mL out.
> - Persevere until you aspirate blood clots.
> - Continue until you have aspirated all blood clots and the catheter is flushing and draining well.

After insertion, don't be alarmed if the patient you were sure had clot retention is now just draining some pink fluid; they could still have a bladder full of clots.

Do a good bladder washout with some sterile water (never use saline). This may take up to 10 minutes of flushing and aspirating, but it is the most important part of the procedure. Bleeding will not stop until you've cleared the bladder of clots.

Ensure you commence irrigation immediately after you have finished the bladder washout otherwise the catheter and bladder will fill with blood clot and all of your hard work will be wasted. You don't want to have to replace that catheter again because it's blocked!

To avoid this always take irrigation fluid with you. If you don't need it (if the urine is draining well and fairly clear), you can always return it.

Common causes
- Post TURP/TURBT. Patients will inevitably be admitted from the day case unit when the surgeon has gone home. Haematuria is to be expected with these procedures. However, frank haematuria or clot retention does require intervention.

- New diagnosis of a malignancy, e.g. bladder or renal (beware the painless haematuria with no apparent cause). These patients will, at some point, require a cystoscopy and renal ultrasound to look for a cause.
- Benign prostatic enlargement (a common cause of many repeat admissions in elderly men, even if they are on finasteride).
- Catheter trauma. Several failed attempts at catheterisation can easily cause bleeding from the prostate especially in those with an enlarged prostate.
- Trauma. This could cause bleeding from any level of the urinary tract and requires investigation. Treat as per ATLS protocol. The management of urological trauma is described in later chapters.
- Urinary tract infection. This is less likely to cause significant prolonged haematuria.

Don't forget . . .

Do a group and save, check a full blood count and treat appropriately

These patients are often elderly, will have little reserve and often a cardiac history. Monitor their haemoglobin and transfuse appropriately. This is especially important if the patient is actively bleeding, as the haemoglobin level on admission is only a snapshot in time.

Check the clotting

Remember to find out if your patient is on warfarin and check the INR. A high INR in an actively bleeding patient needs to be reversed. Depending on your local protocol this may need to be discussed with a haematologist. Be sure to find out why they're on warfarin and check local policies for heparin replacement when the INR is below therapeutic range.

Check renal function

Causes of bleeding such as an enlarged prostate or bladder cancer can also cause obstruction. This can cause impaired renal function that may require urgent intervention such as nephrostomy or ureteric stenting.

Fluid balance

Fluid balance is notoriously difficult in patients on irrigation and non-specialist wards may have trouble with this. Just remember that the output should be greater than the input as the patient should be producing urine on top of the irrigation fluid drained.

Scrotal pain

This is a common surgical referral mainly because primary care and A&E will not want to miss a torsion and therefore request a surgical consult to make that call. You will see many men with scrotal pain. Hardly any of them will have a torsion, but they all require proper assessment. If you are not confident to make this call, then contact your registrar immediately – time is of the essence.

A low threshold of suspicion (in boys) and a fair amount of common sense (in men) will help you. Torsion is most common between 10 and 30 years.

Common causes:
- ⮑ torsion
- ⮑ epididymo-orchitis
- ⮑ hydrocele
- ⮑ torted cyst of Morgagni
- ⮑ epididymal cyst
- ⮑ malignancy.

History and examination

The main objective of this history is determining whether or not there is a torsion. Torsion requires theatre, for everything else there are outpatient clinics.

1 How long has this been going on?
- A torsion that's been going on for days is no longer a surgical emergency. In fact the viability of any torted testicle that's been painful for more than 6 hours is questionable.

2 Pain history
- Is the pain intermittent or constant?

- Are there any exacerbating or relieving factors? A dragging pain from a hydrocele may be relieved when gravity is removed.
- Is there any abdominal pain? A right-sided torsion may well be referred as a suspected appendicitis and is often associated with nausea and vomiting.

3 What were you doing when it started?
- Was it a little boy running around in the playground? Was there any trauma involved (acute hydrocele)? Torsion commonly follows lifting, exercise or masturbation.
- This question is especially helpful in children for establishing a time frame, as they tend to remember things in reference to the school day.
- A gradual onset of pain makes it less likely to be a torsion.

4 Is there any swelling?
- Many of the above causes will cause testicular swelling. Ask yourself, is it actually the testicle or separate from this (epididymal cyst)?
- What's the lie of the testicle? Classically, a torted testicle will sit high in the scrotum with a transverse rather than longitudinal lie. However, this is not always the case, as cremasteric reflex may be absent.

5 Any urinary symptoms or penile discharge?
- Epididymo-orchitis will often start with UTI symptoms.
- It's important to take a sexual history and examine for any lesions on the penis.
- Get a urine dip to check for infection.
- Any patient in which you suspect an STD should be advised to attend the GUM clinic.

> **Common examination findings**
>
> Cremasteric reflex – an upward movement of the testes on stroking the ipsilateral thigh.
>
> Torted cyst of Morgagni – may be visible in a child as a blue spot seen through the scrotum.
>
> Epididymis – this lies posterior to the testicle and may be tender in the case of epididymitis or have a palpable cyst.
>
> Hydrocele – will classically 'light up like a light bulb'. If you can't find a pen torch, the light from an otoscope will do.
>
> Malignancy – this will feel hard and irregular, not like a normal testicle, which should feel like a peeled boiled egg.

Management

Torsion is a surgical emergency and requires exploration in theatre. Don't forget to consent the patient (or parents) for orchidectomy. A torted cyst of Morgagni can usually be left well alone and will resolve. However, many of these patients end up going to theatre for exploration as it is difficult to distinguish clinically from a torsion. It's a brave surgeon who doesn't take a young boy to theatre with acute testicular pain.

Epididymo-orchitis requires antibiotics (check your local guidelines). Most can go home, but if they're systemically unwell they may require admission. Advise rest, scrotal support and simple analgesia. Remember to advise the patient that swelling may take weeks to months to settle completely (many patients re-attend 2 days later because they have not been told this). Scrotal abscess is a recognised complication of epididymo-orchitis and usually presents about a month after the onset of symptoms. If the patient is systemically septic, the abscess will require incision and drainage.

Hydrocele, epididymal cyst or suspected malignancy do not require acute management but may require follow-up in the form of an ultrasound scan and referral for an outpatient appointment (urgently in the case of suspected malignancy).

Renal colic

Suspected renal colic is a common surgical referral. It's usually on the differential for any pain that localises to one particular side. What may be more important is establishing what it's not. Make sure you check for an abdominal aortic aneurysm, as it is not uncommon for these patients to be referred as suffering from renal colic.

History

A good description of the pain is vital here.

- ➲ Is it actually a colicky, intermittent pain?
- ➲ Does it radiate from loin to groin and sometimes into the scrotum in men?
- ➲ Does it make them want to lie still, or roll around as they can't get comfortable? A patient lying perfectly still on the trolley, not wanting to move because of the pain, is unlikely to have renal colic – think peritonitis.
- ➲ Have they had it before? For many patients this will not be their first episode and the pain will be familiar, but you must consider other causes. It's not unheard of to have a renal stone and an aneurysm!

Associated symptoms

- ➲ Are there any urinary symptoms? Stones are a common cause of infection.
- ➲ Are they systemically unwell? An obstructed, infected urinary system may require urgent intervention from a urologist and/or radiologist.

What to do

- ➲ Dip the urine, not only to look for infection but for micro-scopic haematuria – a good indication that something is causing trauma to the urinary tract.

- Check renal function and inflammatory markers.
- X-ray KUB. Whilst the gold standard investigation is CT KUB, this is difficult to get out of hours unless the patient is acutely unwell. CT within 24 hours is acceptable. Sixty per cent of renal tract stones will be visible on a plain X-ray and this will also be useful for comparison in the future (e.g. post treatment).
- Analgesia. Renal colic responds very well to rectal NSAIDs. This may well help with your diagnosis as many renal colic patients are pain-free after PR diclofenac.
- Once you are happy that renal colic is the diagnosis and operative intervention is not required, the patient does not need to be starved. Encourage the patient to drink plenty of water as this may help to flush stones through.

Patients with normal renal function, no sign of infection and whose pain is controlled with simple analgesia can usually go home with an outpatient CT KUB and a referral to the urologist for an outpatient appointment.

When to be worried
- As a general rule of thumb, any stone greater than 6 mm is unlikely to pass by itself and these patients will often require some sort of intervention, either during this admission or electively.

> **Admit for:**
> - analgesia – rectal diclofenac or ketoprofen work well
> - renal impairment – these patients will require IV fluids and, if in acute renal failure, urgent investigation
> - systemic infection – always check inflammatory markers, take blood cultures and start antibiotics early.

➲ An infected, obstructed system will give you an acutely unwell, septic patient who requires close monitoring. Urosepsis can kill patients fast. Check a blood gas if there's any sign of renal impairment and involve ITU early. These patients may require a nephrostomy or ureteric stenting. This may not be done overnight but you should certainly make the urologists aware of the patient.

Phimosis

Phimosis occurs when the foreskin becomes tight and won't retract over the glans penis. This can occur at any age. It is not generally a problem unless the patient is in retention and you need to catheterise.

You'll cause damage if you try to force the foreskin back. Usually a bit of Instillagel® will loosen things up and if you can see the urethral meatus you can catheterise.

How to do a penile block

Sensory innervation to the penis is supplied by the pudendal nerve, which divides into right and left dorsal penile nerves that pass under the pubis symphysis. Attempt to block these nerves as proximally to the base of the penis as possible.

Either: Inject local anaesthetic with one pass at 12 o'clock at the base of the penis and then aim the injection first left and then right of this.

Or: Perform two separate injections at 2 and 10 o'clock on the proximal penile shaft.

This should create a subcutaneous bleb of local anaesthetic. Then insert the needle deeper towards the centre of the shaft to a depth of approximately 0.5 cm. Always aspirate before injecting local anaesthetic (LA) to ensure you're not in a blood vessel. Inject 1–5 mL of LA on both sides depending on patient age, weight and clinical need.

If you can't see the meatus, using an orange needle, inject local anaesthetic (1% lignocaine *without* adrenaline) either as a penile block (see the box below) or circumferentially around the corona of the penis. This will block sensation to the foreskin. The foreskin can then be gently stretched open with a surgical clip. This only needs to be stretched enough to see the external urethral meatus and allow the passage of a catheter. Definitive treatment is elective circumcision.

Paraphimosis

The foreskin gets stuck in a retracted position behind the corona and cannot be easily reduced. This causes oedematous swelling and further tightening. Paraphimosis can be extremely painful and needs to be dealt with quickly as it will only get worse. It can occur at any age but is common in elderly men post-catheterisation, when the foreskin has not been replaced, and young boys.

Management

The treatment is immediate reduction.

- The trick is plenty of lubrication and gentle pressure.
- Have some conversation topics ready as this may take a while.
- Wrap a dry swab around the shaft and hold in one hand.
- Squeeze the glans with a constant pressure; you're trying to get the oedema out.
- As the oedema reduces, you may be able to slip the foreskin back over the glans penis.
- This procedure is neither painless nor pleasant and adequate analgesia is advised. Some patients find that gas and air is sufficient. However, many require oramorph.
- Coating the paraphimosis in sugar or a dextrose-soaked swab may reduce the oedema and aid reduction.
- If you have no success or the patient isn't tolerating further attempts, administer local anaesthetic either as a penile block or circumferentially to the shaft of the penis. This will numb the penis and help your further attempts at reduction. If you are not confident in administering local anaesthetic get your senior to show you. If this fails, the patient will require a dorsal slit (a sagittal incision of the

phimotic ring at 12 o'clock). Again, call your senior if you are not able to do this.

If reduction is successful, the patient can be discharged home with outpatient urology follow-up. Patients often require elective circumcision to prevent further episodes of paraphimosis.

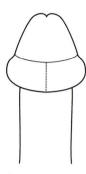

Place clips at the 11 and 1 o'clock positions and incise the foreskin at 12 o'clock.
This will leave a 'V' shaped incision.

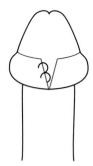

Allow the oedema to ooze out and achieve haemostasis with a simple running stitch using an absorbable suture.

FIGURE 3.2 How to perform a dorsal slit.

Priapism

This is a persistent, painful erection of more than 4 hours' duration in the absence of sexual desire. You may think it sounds hilarious, but have some sympathy; your patient will be in pain and embarrassed. If left untreated, it can result in ischaemic damage to the penis and permanent erectile dysfunction. Patients often present late due to embarrassment. It is important to quantify the duration of erection.

Priapism is usually idiopathic, but establish whether there is any underlying or secondary cause such as:

- ➲ intracavernosal injection therapy (penile injections patients are prescribed for erectile dysfunction)
- ➲ other medications (many drugs can cause this, so just take a thorough drug history)
- ➲ sickle cell disease, leukaemia, thalassaemia (due to small thrombo-embolic events)
- ➲ neurological conditions such as spinal cord lesions and autonomic neuropathy (beware the trauma patient with priapism; it's a sign of neurogenic shock)
- ➲ penile or perineal trauma causing disruption to the penile arterial supply.

Priapism is classified as either low-flow (ischaemic) or high-flow (non-ischaemic) priapism:

> **Low-flow priapism:**
> - ◕ most common type
> - ◕ due to venous occlusion
> - ◕ painful rigid erection
> - ◕ blood gas analysis aspirated from the penile corpora shows hypoxia and acidosis.

> **High-flow priapism:**
> - less common
> - due to abnormal arterial flow
> - painless, semi-rigid erection
> - blood gas analysis aspirated from the penile corpora is normal (i.e. similar to ABG).

Low-flow priapism of duration greater than 4 hours requires emergency intervention. High-flow priapism is usually self-limiting and does not require emergency intervention.

Management of low-flow (ischaemic) priapism

- The aim is to try and divert blood flow away from the penis. Get your patient to exercise, jogging up and down stairs, press-ups, jumping, whatever they can do. They will have to exercise vigorously for at least 20 minutes, but if this works it has saved the need for further intervention.
- Ice packs on the penis may reduce the erection.
- If this doesn't work then you may have to drain the blood manually. If you are not confident doing this, then call your registrar.
- If manual drainage fails, the patient will need an intra-cavernosal injection of phenylephrine. You should call your registrar to do this. Patients require continuous cardiac monitoring during intracavernosal phenylephrine injection. You can help by arranging a suitable place for this to be done, such as A&E resus. If this fails, they will need surgical intervention organised by your registrar.

Manual drainage

Clean the penis with iodine prep.

Create a skin bleb with 1–2 mL 1% lignocaine *without* adrenaline on either lateral aspect of the penis roughly at the mid-shaft.

Through the anaesthetised areas insert a green or larger sized butterfly needle into the penis and allow the blood to drain into two kidney dishes, one on either side of the penis. You need to allow free flow of blood into the dishes until oxygenated red blood is observed.

If the erection is still present after 10 minutes, try flushing normal saline into the penis through the butterfly needles, 5 mL either side at a time. Essentially 'watering down' the concentration of blood in the corpora cavernosum may reduce the erection.

Urological trauma

Urological trauma is uncommon. Unlike trauma to other intra-abdominal structures it often doesn't require emergency intervention. However, in any trauma patient ensure you have looked for possible urological trauma. This requires a good secondary survey and a urine dip.

Renal trauma

The kidneys are well protected in the retroperitoneum, so are rarely damaged even in severe trauma cases. However, loin pain and haematuria in a patient with a history of trauma should not be ignored. It will not always be high-energy trauma; you may be called to see the old lady who's had a fall, the teenager who's been playing rugby or the woman who's been hit by a shopping trolley (yes, it's happened!).

Renal trauma is classified as grades 1–5 on CT imaging. Almost all renal trauma is managed conservatively (grades 1–4). Only grade 5 injuries, a completely shattered kidney or an avulsion of the renal hilum, need urgent surgical intervention. If the kidney has been this badly injured, the patient is highly likely to have other organ damage (spleen, liver, etc.) and require immediate laparotomy. This patient will be shocked. If the patient is haemodynamically unstable, has a drop in their haemoglobin or has persistent frank haematuria, call your registrar, as they will need out-of-hours imaging and possible intervention.

Haemodynamically stable patients, with minimal decrease in haemoglobin and microscopic haematuria or one or two episodes of self-limiting frank haematuria, do not need urgent imaging if they present out of hours. Admit them for strict bed rest, site two large-bore IV cannulas and request a group and save. A CT scan can be performed the next morning allowing further management to be planned.

Ureteric trauma

This is usually iatrogenic due to pelvic or abdominal surgery and dealt with at the time. Rarely it may be due to blunt or penetrating trauma. This does not need immediate intervention.

Bladder trauma

Bladder trauma is usually iatrogenic due to pelvic or abdominal surgery and dealt with at the time. It is often associated with trauma that causes pelvic fractures and associated urethral injuries may be present. Blood at the external urethral meatus suggests a urethral injury. Presentation may be with suprapubic pain, haematuria and difficulty voiding. If the patient is having CT imaging, ask the radiologist to check for bladder or urethral injuries. This may require a separate urethrogram and cystogram to be performed. Bladder injury may be extra- or intraperitoneal.

Extraperitoneal injury

Usual type associated with pelvic fractures. Urine escapes into space around bladder but not into peritoneum. Treat with open surgical repair only if associated injuries require surgical repair or if there is a need to place a suprapubic catheter via open surgery (such as an associated urethral injury contraindicating urethral catheterisation). If surgery is not required, insert either urethral or suprapubic catheter and leave for 10 days. Remove only after a cystogram has confirmed no urine leak.

> **Intraperitoneal injury**
>
> Usually associated with direct blow to a distended full bladder (i.e. seat belt/steering wheel/fall), causing a sudden rise in intravesical pressure and hence rupture. Urine escapes into peritoneal cavity, causing abdominal pain, abdominal distension, absent bowel sounds and an associated ileus. Requires immediate surgical repair.

Urethral trauma

Urethral trauma is very uncommon in women. In men, either posterior or anterior injuries can occur. Posterior urethral injury is commonly associated with pelvic fractures. Anterior urethral injury is uncommon and associated with a straddle injury. Both types present with blood at the external urethral meatus, haematuria and have difficulty voiding. Bruising of the scrotum, penis, perineum and abdomen may occur if Buck's fascia has been ruptured. Urethral trauma is diagnosed by retrograde urethrogram.

All urethral injuries are best treated with suprapubic catheterisation to divert urine flow, and elective surgical treatment when swelling has subsided. If the patient is in retention, then suprapubic catheterisation can be easily performed. If the patient is not in retention, wait for the urology team to place a suprapubic catheter during daylight hours.

Testicular trauma

Patients will present with a history of trauma and a bruised and swollen scrotum. The scrotum will be acutely tender and the testicle is unlikely to be palpable due to a surrounding haematoma. You need to get a testicular USS to look for testicular rupture. This can wait until daylight hours. If the USS shows a scrotal haematoma and no rupture, this can be treated conservatively. If a rupture is present, surgical repair is required.

Fractured penis

This is usually a result of rigorous sexual activity. Injury occurs when the erect penis is forced into the female bony pubis, resulting in rupture of the tunica albuginea of the penis. Patients report a snapping sound followed by immediate loss of erection, penile pain and subsequent penile bruising. Bruising and swelling is significant and the penis is often said to look like an aubergine. You must check for associated urethral damage.

If the patient is in retention, they require catheterisation. Due to the risk of urethral injury it's best to only attempt a urethral catheter once. If unsuccessful, site a suprapubic catheter. If the patient is voiding and it's out of hours, the patient needs to be admitted for analgesia and kept nil by mouth, so that the urology team can arrange surgical repair. Ensure you hand over to the urology day team early so that this can be organised. Surgical repair is recommended within 24 hours of fracture. Late presentation does not require surgery but will require follow-up with urology.

Catheters

Many inpatients require catheterisation and many referrals to hospital are due to catheter-related problems. As the surgical junior on call, you will frequently be called to troubleshoot catheter problems. Having some basic catheter knowledge and knowing how to deal with catheter problems will certainly make your shift less stressful.

Catheters:

⮡ range from 12 (small) to 28 (large) French
⮡ are either male or female in length
⮡ have a maximum insertion time of 3 weeks (short term – usually PTFE orange/brown soft catheter) or 12 weeks (long term – usually silicone clear stiffer catheter), depending on the catheter material
⮡ can be two-way (two ports – one for urine drainage, one for inflating the balloon) or three-way (three ports – as for two-way but with an extra port for instilling irrigating fluid into the bladder)
⮡ are held intravesically with a balloon. Always inflate the balloon with sterile water – *do not use anything else*. Always inflate with 10 mL, except three-way catheters, which should take 20–30 mL. Always document how much water you used to inflate the balloon so the person removing the catheter knows how much water to extract.

Urethral catheter problems

Difficult male catheterisation

Sometimes, however much you might want it to, it just won't go in. Here are a few tips to help you keep your calm and avoid that embarrassing call to the registrar.

⮡ Liberal use of Instillagel®. The volume of the male urethral is 20 mL so you can use two tubes. This is always recommended when inserting a three-way catheter.

- ↻ Hold the penis upright to keep the urethra straight. Remember your anatomy and the position of the prostate. When the catheter hits the prostate, lower the penis to the bed between the patient's legs.
- ↻ If you feel resistance at the prostate/sphincter, ask the patient to relax as if passing urine or coughing.
- ↻ Gentle pressure when you hit the obstruction will help (don't just jab at it, you'll create a false passage).
- ↻ Short-term PTFE catheters are soft and may buckle on hitting the prostate. Try a stiffer long-term catheter that may slip past the prostate rather than buckle. Better still try a Coudé tip or Tiemann tip catheter. These have a slight curvature at the tip, which is designed to follow the anatomy of the prostate. They are very effective and your life will be infinitely easier if you know where these are kept. Just remember to keep the curve facing up when placing it.

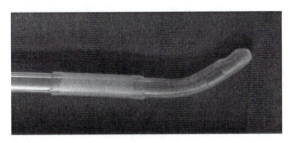

FIGURE 3.3 The tip of a Coudé tip catheter, which is curved to better pass the prostate.

Difficult female catheterisation

Most nurses are competent in female catheterisation so you will rarely get asked to perform this on the wards. When you do get called it will be because they have failed. Female catheterisation is easy so don't be fazed. The problem is most commonly that the external urethral meatus is difficult to locate. In some women it is located high up in the introitus hiding behind the clitoris. You may need to get the patient towards the edge of the bed whilst you get down on your knees to look up and locate it! Usually it is because the woman is obese and it is difficult to get good exposure. The key is good lighting and a helpful assistant. You may need one or more nurses to help spread the patient's legs and vulva, leaving you with free hands to catheterise. Ensure the patient is lying flat otherwise you will be fighting against their abdomen!

Painful catheter

You may be asked to review a patient complaining of catheter-related pain. There are many reasons for this pain. The most important is that the catheter has been sited incorrectly. A catheter balloon inflated in the urethra will cause significant pain and the patient will report this immediately. If this history is absent and the catheter is draining, then it is most likely in the correct place. Check by making sure that the catheter flushes well with no pain to the patient. If you are still unsure, you can check the catheter position by deflating the balloon, pushing the catheter in further and re-inflating the balloon. If you still have any doubts about the position of the catheter, remove it and re-insert a new catheter.

If you are confident the catheter is in correctly, try and ascertain where the patient is experiencing pain. Men often complain of penile pain secondary to catheter irritation. This can be treated with PRN topical Instillagel®. Another cause of penile pain may be due to irritation from the catheter balloon rubbing on the trigone of the bladder. Trigonal irritation is often felt as penile pain. If the patient complains of intermittent spasms of suprapubic pain, this is most likely to be due to bladder spasm. These are bladder muscle contractions against the catheter balloon. These can be excruciating for the patient but are easily treated with an anti-cholinergic drug, such as oxybutynin 2.5 mg tds or solifenacin 5 mg od.

Catheter not draining

The catheter is either blocked, in the wrong place or the patient is not producing urine. You can work out which by examining the patient: Are they in retention? Is the catheter causing them pain? What is their fluid balance? What is their renal function? Once again, simple measures like palpating the abdomen, performing a bladder scan and flushing the catheter will help you decide what needs to be done. If you are still unsure, change the catheter.

Bypassing catheters

Bypassing catheters is a common issue on the medical ward. Usually it is a long-term catheter that is blocked with debris and either needs changing or a flush.
- Always flush with sterile water and aspirate what you put in.
- When this doesn't work just try changing it. It won't hurt to go up a size; this will help with drainage and make the catheter less likely to clog in the future.

Bleeding

Whether it's due to repeated attempts at catheterisation or

the balloon being inflated too early, you will often be the first call when someone is now, unsurprisingly, bleeding from their prostate.

- ➲ Don't panic. Unless they are on warfarin and haemorrhaging, it will stop.
- ➲ Put into practice your newly acquired catheter skills and calmly amaze them with your competence.
- ➲ As long as the catheter is draining, you do not need to do anything. Catheter-related bleeding will hopefully settle. If the catheter blocks with clot or there is persistent frank haematuria, you will need to change the catheter to a three-way and commence irrigation.
- ➲ Make sure you enquire as to how many attempts have been made. Repeated attempts, especially ones that cause bleeding, may need to be covered with a shot of antibiotics to prevent urosepsis (check your local guidelines).

Suprapubic catheters

Do not site a new suprapubic catheter by yourself, unless you have been trained and are confident you can do so. People are often panicked by suprapubic catheters, especially if blocked and bypassing. However, with no prostate in the way, they couldn't be easier to deal with.

Changing is a simple job, and realistically any doctor or nurse should be able to do this.

- ➲ The most important thing to remember is that the tract can disappear within hours, especially if the catheter is new. Once removed, replace as quickly as possible.
- ➲ Simply deflate the balloon and withdraw the catheter. If blocked and the patient is in retention, stand back and have something handy to prevent a puddle of urine.
- ➲ Proceed as you would a normal catheterisation. The

only difference being that you do not want to push the catheter all the way in, as you would a urethral catheter, before inflating the balloon. It's not unheard of for the tip to pass right through the bladder and out of the urethra, especially in women. The tract formed by a suprapubic catheter will only be a few centimetres.

- ➲ If the tract has closed and you cannot replace the suprapubic catheter, insert a urethral catheter and refer the patient to urology for elective suprapubic re-insertion.

Difficulty removing a catheter

Occasionally you may be called to a catheter that will not come out. This is usually due to a balloon that won't deflate. Try the following steps one by one until you are successful.

1 Ensure the balloon is within the bladder by pushing it in further before attempting further deflation.
2 Inject 1 mL of water into the balloon before trying to deflate the balloon slowly. If you try to deflate it too quickly, the valve mechanism will collapse.
3 Remove the plunger from a syringe and insert the remaining syringe into the catheter balloon port. Leave for 5 minutes. This opens the balloon to the atmosphere and with time it may deflate slowly.
4 Cut the balloon port off with scissors. Make sure you do this distal to where it separates from the main catheter, otherwise the catheter may retract into the urethra. Cutting the balloon port will allow the water to drain from the balloon spontaneously.
5 Insert a ureteric guidewire up through the balloon port in an attempt to pop the balloon. You will be able to get a ureteric guidewire from theatres. Dispose in the sharps bin after use.

6   Ask the radiologist to perform ultrasound-guided suprapu-
    bic balloon puncture.
7   Call the urologist!

If it is out of hours and your attempts at steps 1–5 have failed, leave the catheter in and steps 6 or 7 can be sorted out in the morning. You may be lucky and find that by morning the catheter has eventually fallen out on mobilising the patient and the balloon has simply taken hours to deflate.

Chapter 4

ENT

Ven Reddy and
Warren Bennett

Epistaxis

Epistaxis can be life-threatening and should be taken very seriously. History should be direct and quick, as treatment often needs to be prompt. Features of the onset of bleeding should be ascertained. Most bleeds originate anteriorly, but if it started at the back of the mouth a posterior bleeding point may be the cause. Significant hypertension may make it harder to control the bleeding and might require treatment. The drug history may reveal the use of anticoagulants such as clopidogrel and warfarin. Depending on the indication, these anticoagulants may need to be stopped or their effects reversed. Past medical history may reveal coagulopathies that need to be addressed. A relevant medical condition to identify is hereditary haemorrhagic telangiectasia, in which abnormal blood vessel formation can cause frequent epistaxis and gastrointestinal bleeding. These patients, and their families, are often known to the department and they may tell you what has worked for them in the past!

Preparation is everything. You need to be suitably protected, as there is a chance that blood will be spat and coughed everywhere. You need to have eye protection, mask, gloves and an apron. As with everything serious in medicine, the approach should always be ABC. The airway should be cleared of clot using suction and/or Magill's forceps. Large-bore IV access should be established with appropriate fluid resuscitation. Bloods should be taken including a group and save, or cross-match if appropriate, full blood count and coagulation screen.

Begin with the basics – simple pressure may halt the deluge! Get the patient or a willing helper to pinch the soft fleshy part of the nose firmly for 15 minutes continuously. Pinching for a short amount of time may be ineffective and pinching the hard bony part of the nose will achieve nothing.

The patient should lean forwards not backwards, as they will ingest large amounts of blood, which will most likely lead to vomiting. Ice packs can be applied to the back of the neck and over the dorsum of the nose, or the patient could suck on some ice cubes to encourage vasoconstriction. This may give them a headache but it's a favourable alternative to continuing haemorrhage.

Whilst this is all being done, you can plan your next move. If the bleeding has stopped, you need to have a look in the nose to see if you can identify a point in the nose that may benefit from cautery. To do this you will need a good headlight and a Thudicum nasal speculum to get a good view. Ask the patient to gently blow their nose to clear any clots. Suction can be used to remove blood clots (a Yankauer sucker for big anterior clots, and a Zoellner sucker for smaller ones). Apply local anaesthetic/vasoconstrictor (e.g. lignocaine with phenylephrine) soaked on a bit of cotton wool ball. This is inserted using a Tilley's dressing forceps and pressed for several minutes over the area to be cauterised.

The most commonly available cautery device is the silver nitrate stick. Once you have identified the bleeding point, apply the tip of the cautery stick working in a spiral direction around the bleeding point working towards the middle. If there is a scab over the bleeding point, this should be removed first. After cautery, prescribe a nasal ointment to keep the cauterised area moist. The ointments have antibacterial properties, as a localised low-grade infection may have a role in some patients. Such ointments include Naseptin (peanut oil based) and Bactroban. In children with recurrent brief episodes of epistaxis, it is appropriate to try this in the first instance (e.g. Naseptin to be applied twice a day for 3 weeks). Where chronic nasal dryness is a precipitant, regular application of simple petroleum jelly may be useful. Patients should be advised to avoid straining, stooping or any vigorous exercise as this may aggravate bleeding. Traditionally, patients have been advised to avoid ingesting hot food or drinks for several days, but there is little evidence for the benefits of this.

If there is active bleeding, apply local anaesthetic/vasoconstrictor as previously described. Hopefully, this will reduce the bleeding and make it suitable for cautery. If the bleeding remains severe, the process can be repeated before cautery is attempted. Beware of the amount of medication you use.

It is important to adjust other factors that may help control the bleeding, namely clotting and blood pressure. If clotting is abnormal and reversal is safe (e.g. an INR well beyond therapeutic range where there is a soft indication for warfarin), then it should be considered. If the patient has a known coagulopathy, this must be corrected otherwise your interventions are less likely to succeed. A high systolic blood pressure may hinder your efforts to control the bleeding. Seek medical advice if you are unsure.

The next step in management is nasal packing. There are several different types of nasal packs but most work by tamponade effect. Some have a gelatinous coating that needs to be activated with sterile water, so check the instructions. The patient must be warned that it will be unpleasant, and analgesia should be offered. The pack is inserted horizontally along the floor of the nose (not into the roof of the nose), and should be placed in entirety (not half hanging out) though occasionally septal deviation may make this difficult to achieve. Support the back of the head with one hand and insert the pack with the other hand along the floor of the nose. Do this swiftly as it is less uncomfortable overall. After a few minutes, if this manages to stop the bleeding, the oropharynx should be checked to make sure there is no active bleeding posteriorly. The patient is admitted for observation and the pack is removed after 24 hours. If the bleeding continues, the contralateral side can also be packed to apply counter pressure. If the patient is still bleeding, posterior packing should be considered. Unless you have been trained or have been shown, you should get senior assistance for posterior packing.

If the bleeding cannot be controlled, call your seniors for help. They may want to inspect the nose themselves for a bleeding point. If they too are unsuccessful, surgical options will need to be implemented such as septoplasty and/or endoscopic ligation of the sphenopalatine artery.

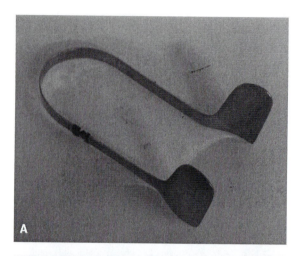

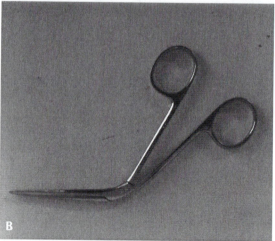

FIGURE 4.1 Useful ENT equipment: (a) Thudichum speculum, (b) Nasal Tilley's forceps, (c) Wax hook, (d) Jobson-Horne probe, (e) Silver nitrate nasal cautery stick, (f) Nasal pack – Rapid Rhino, (g) Nasal pack – Merocel.

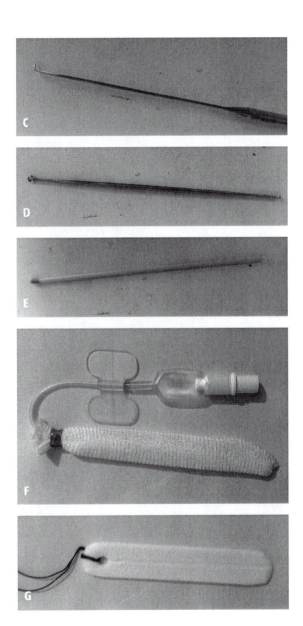

Foreign bodies and food boluses

If the foreign body (FB) is a battery, it must be removed immediately! Call your senior straight away.

Ear

These should be removed under the microscope to give you a good view because of the risk of pushing them deeper, injuring the ear canal wall and perforating the eardrum.

The method of removal depends on the shape of the FB. A spherical object that is not filling the ear canal can be removed by getting the end of a wax hook behind it and drawing it out. If a spherical object is filling the ear canal wall, you can try using microsuction. FBs with an edge to grab hold of can be removed using crocodile forceps.

Water must not be used for certain objects that absorb water, such as sponges or seeds as they will expand causing pain and making removal more difficult. Syringing with warm water is an option for non-organic matter only and in patients without a history of tympanic membrane perforation. Fill a syringe with warm water (check the temperature on yourself and the parent or patient). Pull the pinna back and direct the tip of the syringe up to the roof of the ear canal before injecting. The water should get behind the FB and push it out. Get an assistant to hold a kidney dish next to the ear as you do this or you will get wet! Topical antibiotics can be prescribed if there is evidence of infection. Live insects should be drowned with olive oil then removed with microsuction. Hopefully the insect will be removed whole otherwise you will have to pick it out piecemeal!

With children, if you are not confident in removing the FB, make arrangements for the child to return when senior ENT support is available, as children do not give you many attempts. Do not cause the child undue distress. A quick general anaesthetic may be more appropriate on the next elective list, if it is not weeks away!

Nose

These are of more concern as they are technically in the airway. Longstanding nasal FBs may present with a purulent or bloody nasal discharge. Some FBs may have dislodged, been exhaled or swallowed by the time you see them despite what an anxious parent may tell you. Using a headlight, the tip of the nose is lifted and this may reveal the problem. The otoscope with speculum offers some magnification, which may help. The 'kissing technique' uses the parent to dislodge the foreign body by getting them to blow into the child's mouth whilst blocking the unobstructed nostril. For direct removal, a child can be kept still by getting them to sit on their parent's lap, with the parent putting one of their hands across the child's forehead and the other arm across the child's arms and chest or alternatively wrapped in a blanket. Use an earwax hook or Jobson-Horne probe with a curved end to get over and behind the FB then draw it out. If the FB has an edge, a crocodile forcep may be more successful. If there is some bleeding, infection or the FB has been in for a while, prescribe Naseptin or Bactroban cream to be applied 2 times a day for 2 weeks.

If the patient is not cooperating, remember there is a theoretical risk of aspirating the FB, so admit the patient and have them starved ready for a short general anaesthetic the next day. Explain to the parents that the ENT team may want to try removal again before definitely resorting to theatre.

Throat

Bones in fish and meat or sharp objects can become impaled in the throat. Patients often cannot localise the site where the FB resides. A thorough examination will in most cases establish whether there is an FB or just mucosal abrasion. Lateral soft tissue neck X-rays will show up radiopaque FBs but can be difficult to interpret due to variable calcification of cartilages and blood vessels, depending on the age of the patient. Things that will not show up on X-ray are plastic, aluminium and certain fish bones (herring, mackerel, salmon, skate and trout). We recommend examination using a Mackintosh laryngoscope, as it has a light and a curved shape that lends itself to looking at the tonsils, base of the tongue and vallecula (the most common sites for FBs to become impaled). With the patient sat up, use the Mackintosh laryngoscope to press down on the tongue. Work your way backwards to ensure you do not miss anything. If the patient has a strong gag reflex or doesn't tolerate examination well, use xylocaine spray to numb the base of tongue and the throat. If the patient keeps moving their head away from you, get them to lie on a couch with their head slightly extended over the edge and re-examine (as an anaesthetist would to intubate). Perform a fiberoptic nasendoscopy and ask the patient to do a valsalva to splint the pyriform fossae open. Most FBs can be removed with a Magill's forceps. Bones impaled below the base of tongue might need removal under general anaesthesia.

If you cannot see any foreign body on examination or on lateral neck X-ray, and you have a low index of suspicion (e.g. the patient is well, afebrile, able to swallow) reassure the patient that their symptoms are most likely due to an abrasion. If this is the case, it should resolve within a few days. If their symptoms worsen they should return for reassessment. If you have a high index of suspicion and the patient is well, ask your seniors to review the patient. If it is the middle of the night, this can wait until the next day. If you have a high index of suspicion and the patient is unwell (e.g. severe pain, febrile, drooling, unable to swallow, etc.) admit the patient and inform your senior. Fine fish bones are less worrying than hard bones from meat and chicken, which have a higher risk of perforation and should be removed urgently.

Children often put objects in their mouths that may end up in the airway or the oesophagus. An AP and lateral neck X-ray will demonstrate this if the FB is radiopaque (coins are popular). A history of a brief coughing fit followed by stridor may suggest FB in the airway (*see* 'Acute stridor', pp. 97–100). A chest X-ray should be performed as this may demonstrate an FB in the lower respiratory tract and lung collapse due to bronchial obstruction. Absolute dysphagia, painful swallowing and drooling may be associated with an FB stuck in the cricopharyngeus or oesophagus. These need urgent removal, so call your senior.

Food bolus

If a food bolus contains bone, obtain a lateral neck soft tissue X-ray. This needs urgent removal, as there is a risk of oesophageal perforation. Call your senior for review and further management.

With soft food, boluses establish whether the obstruction is partial or complete, which may be indicated by whether they are able to swallow their own saliva or not. Ask the patient to try to sip some water. If it goes down comfortably and stays down, proceed to a soft diet, which if tolerated will give you confidence that there is no food bolus. If the water goes down but with discomfort the patient may have a partial obstruction. If the water is thrown up immediately, it suggests a high obstruction. If the water is thrown up after a delay, it suggests a lower obstruction.

Soft food boluses may resolve spontaneously, so conservative management is appropriate for up to 24 hours. Admit the patient and if they are able to swallow fluids, try carbonated drinks such as cola initially. Remember to keep nil by mouth from midnight in case an anaesthetic is needed. Administer buscopan 20 mg IM repeated after 30 minutes and diazepam 5 mg IV. Reassess the next day; if it is felt to be a high obstruction, the patient is best dealt with by ENT surgeons using rigid oesophagoscopy. If it is more likely to be a low obstruction, it is more safely dealt with by the gastroenterologists using flexible OGD.

Acute stridor

Stridor most commonly refers to high-pitched noisy breathing due to turbulent airflow through a partially obstructed airway at or below the larynx. The nature of the stridor therefore provides clues about the level of airway obstruction.

- ➲ Inspiratory – supraglottic or glottic obstruction.
- ➲ Inspiratory and expiratory (biphasic) – glottic or subglottic obstruction.
- ➲ Expiratory – tracheo-bronchial obstruction.

Stertor on the other hand is a low-pitched noisy breathing, like snoring, indicating obstruction above the larynx.

There are many causes of stridor, both chronic and acute, but this section will focus on providing you with an approach to dealing with an acute stridor. A compromised airway can progress quickly – call your seniors as soon as you are referred a case of suspected stridor – they will want to know about these patients as soon as possible. Quietening stridor may not be an improvement – it may indicate tiring respiratory effort or severe hypercapnia.

Rapid assessment is necessary involving elements of history, examination and intervention simultaneously. The patient should be assessed and managed in the resus bays.

LOOK: alertness, colour (blue = bad), respiratory rate, oxygen sats, use of accessory muscles of respiration (tracheal tug, intercostal recession, etc.), tongue (swelling suggests angioedema or floor of mouth cellulitis) .

LISTEN: is the stridor inspiratory/expiratory/both? Is there a cough? Is the patient talking in full sentences/partial sentences/words/less (indicates alertness and tiredness)?

The history will give you some clues as to the underlying pathology:

- ⊃ onset (immediate = anaphylaxis/foreign body, hours = infection/inflammation, days/weeks = neoplastic)
- ⊃ associated symptoms (pain/odynophagia = inflammation/ infection, barking cough = croup, feverish = infection)
- ⊃ in children, a brief coughing fit preceding stridor may suggest a foreign body in the airway.

Immediate treatment: general principles (except epiglottitis, see below)

If the patient is hypoxic administer high flow O_2 via face mask or nasal prongs. If available in your department, Heliox may be a useful alternative (a mixture of helium and oxygen, which is less viscous than air and therefore gets past airway obstructions to the lungs more effectively). Nebulised adrenaline 1 mL of 1:1000 adrenaline in 5 mL of normal saline will buy you time as the vasoconstriction reduces oedema and can be repeated once the effects wear off if necessary. IV dexamethasone (8 mg in adults, 300 mg/kg in children) helps reduce inflammation. If infection is suspected (supraglottitis/epiglottitis) prescribe intravenous ceftriaxone 2 g BD (adult dose).

If the airway is stable (responded to treatment, not deteriorating), the patient can go to an ENT ward or an HDU with nurses experienced in monitoring and managing airway compromise. Don't admit the patient to an alternative ward where the required expertise is missing. If you are concerned that the airway is not stable, you must also call the ICU and anaesthetic team immediately, as the patient may require close monitoring in an ITU environment with possible intubation to secure the airway. Investigations depend on the suspected cause. Never send a patient with an unstable airway away for an investigation. In adults, a fiberoptic examination is useful to establish the diagnosis – if you know what you're looking for.

As well as the above general management, specific management varies with different causes, e.g. epiglottitis, croup, angioeneurotic oedema, hereditary angioneurotic oedema, Ludwig's angina and neoplastic lesions.

Epiglottitis

This is rare nowadays thanks to the Haemophilus influenzae type B (Hib) vaccine, but it does still occur in both children and adults. Children will present with stridor, tachypnoea, looking unwell, drooling, sitting upright and using accessory muscles of breathing. Don't do anything that may distress the child. Inform senior ENT, anaesthetic, paediatrics doctors and the theatre team, as further management should take place in the theatre environment. The anaesthetic team will try to intubate the child to secure the airway. The child will then remain on ITU receiving IV antibiotics and steroids for 24–48 hours before extubation is attempted. If the anaesthetist is unable to secure the airway, the ENT surgeon will become involved.

Croup (laryngotracheobronchitis)

Children are usually affected, but occasionally adults too. Croup is mostly due to a viral infection, but as it may also be bacterial, treatment is with antibiotics (IV ceftriaxone). The classic presentation is with pyrexia, inspiratory or biphasic stridor and a 'barking' cough. The child should be admitted to a paediatric HDU for observation.

Angioeneurotic oedema

Features are swelling of the tongue, mucous membranes

and face. This is most commonly acquired secondary to ACE-inhibitor use. Stop the ACE-inhibitor! Treatment includes IV dexamethasone (8 mg) and chlorpheniramine (10 mg), +/– nebulised adrenaline (1 mL of 1 : 1000 in 5 mL normal saline).

Hereditary angioneurotic oedema

This is rare, not associated with ACE-Inhibitors, anaphylactic triggers or a family history and does not respond to steroids/antihistamine. It is associated with complement dysfunction (C1 esterase inhibitor deficiency), and C4 and C2 levels will need to be checked – if low, C1 esterase inhibitor levels will then be checked. Treatment is with fresh frozen plasma.

Ludwig's angina

This is cellulitis of the floor of the mouth, which is associated with pyrexia and drooling. This is usually due to dental infection – get an orthopantomogram (OPG) X-ray and ask the maxillofacial surgeons to review. If the source is a dental abscess, it will need drainage urgently. Commence IV augmentin 1.2 g TDS if not contraindicated, analgesia and IV fluids.

Neoplastic lesions

These should always be considered in a patient with risk factors (smokers/drinkers >50 years) and a gradually worsening hoarse voice, stridor and dyspnoea. A CT scan and senior review will be required.

Tonsillitis

Tonsillitis is a common ENT emergency. It is most commonly viral initially but may be complicated by bacterial infection. Severely affected patients will be unable to swallow due to pain and are at risk of dehydration. Complications of tonsillitis are quinsy (peritonsillar abscess), deep neck space infections and, rarely, airway obstruction (due to grossly enlarged tonsils usually secondary to infectious mononucleosis).

History

Tonsillitis is characterised by sore throat, painful swallowing (odynophagia), fever, malaise and a muffled voice ('hot potato' voice).

Examination

Use a good light and a tongue depressor to get a decent view of the tonsils. Tonsillitis often demonstrates a cellulitic appearance of the peritonsillar area, the tonsils are usually enlarged and they will often have a white covering (exudate). There may be associated enlarged and tender lymph nodes in the upper neck. Pharyngitis and other infections of the pharynx and larynx should not be confused with tonsillitis, which is quite distinct.

When to admit

The key to whether the patient needs admission is whether they are able to swallow. If they can swallow, they can take oral antibiotics, analgesia and fluids without the need for admission. If they cannot swallow, they will need admission for IV antibiotics, IV analgesia and IV fluids.

General treatment principles

If the patient is being admitted, and there are no contraindications, use IV benzylpenicillin +/- IV metronidazole. If the patient is sensitive to penicillin, discuss with microbiology as local prescribing practices vary (cefuroxime or a macrolide might be appropriate). A dose of corticosteroid can help reduce oedema, inflammation and pain. In adults, 4–8 mg of dexamethasone is given if there are no contraindications. Patients will often improve vastly after 24–48 hours. At this point they can be switched to oral antibiotics, normally to complete a 7-day course. Patients recover at different rates, so they should be informed to resume normal activities as their recovery permits.

If the patient is not being admitted, a 7–10 day course of oral antibitotics (penicillin V +/– metronidazole) and analgesia (paracetamol and ibuprofen) should be prescribed.

Investigations

For patients that are admitted, a full blood count and CRP are helpful. The FBC may reveal a neutrophilia consistent with bacterial infection. A lymphocytosis may suggest infectious mononucleosis.

Aftercare

For an isolated uncomplicated episode of tonsillitis, follow-up is not indicated. However, follow-up should be considered if a patient has had multiple admissions to hospital for tonsillitis, or two or more episodes of quinsy. Arrange an outpatient follow-up to discuss tonsillectomy. This will allow the patient to be appropriately consented and processed through the hospital's preoperative preparation pathways. Current SIGN guidelines recommend that tonsillectomy is otherwise only performed when patients have 7 or more confirmed cases of tonsillitis in 1 year, 5 each year for 2 years, or 3 a year for 3 years. If the above criteria are not met, patients should be advised to see their GP when they have a sore throat, as they will monitor it and refer if appropriate.

Associated pathologies

Infectious mononucleosis (glandular fever)

Infectious mononucleosis is associated with Epstein-Barr virus infection. A lymphocytosis on the differential white cell count may suggest this. Monospot or Paul Bunnell test should be performed if infectious mononucleosis is suspected. If the test comes back negative but you still suspect clinically that the patient has glandular fever, then the test should be repeated in the near future as the test does have a high false-negative rate in the first 1–2 weeks of illness. LFTs should also be checked as they may be deranged. It is important to identify glandular fever as the patient needs to be informed that this is a viral illness that will last for several weeks and that they should avoid contact sports for 12 weeks as the associated hepatosplenomegaly puts them at risk of significant injury following relatively minor blunt trauma. Even though it is a viral condition, antibiotics are commonly used in glandular fever, as there may be a superimposed bacterial infection. Amoxicillin/co-amoxiclav should not be used as this can cause a scarring rash in patients with glandular fever.

Quinsy/peritonsillar abscess

This is a complication of tonsillitis in which a collection forms between the tonsil and the adjacent tonsil bed. Patients will usually complain of unilateral throat pain (bilateral quinsy is extremely rare), pyrexia, deviation of the uvula to the opposite side, trismus (limited jaw opening due to spasm in the muscles of mastication) and a protruding soft palate. On many occasions a patient will be referred with a suspected quinsy due to pain or tonsillar swelling that is worse on one side with none of the signs discussed, in which case quinsy is less likely. Treatment is the same as any abscess – drain it! This can be performed by aspiration using a 10–20 mL syringe (use the largest syringe that the patient's mouth opening will allow), and a large-bore needle (16 g or 18 g). If you are not confident doing this, discuss this with your senior. If the patient arrives in the middle of the night, admit them for analgesia and leave it for the next day when somebody can supervise you doing it.

If you are able to attempt aspiration, explain the procedure to the patient: it is not pleasant but draining the pus should aid recovery. Explain that your efforts may be unsuccessful, and that there is a possibility of recollection after successful aspiration, which may require further drainage. Use a good light and tongue depressor, spray the throat with xylocaine spray, advise the patient to gargle the anaesthetic for as long as is comfortable before either swallowing it or spitting it out. After a few minutes allowing the topical anaesthetic to work, insert the needle as indicated in Figure 4.2 whilst pulling the plunger back. Hopefully the syringe will fill with pus and the patient will often get instant relief! Don't go too deep or too laterally – there is a big blood vessel nearby! If the quinsy recollects, the ENT team may perform incision and drainage using a scalpel.

Depending on the patient and your hospital policy, some will need admission and others often just a single shot of IV antibiotics +/– steroids. Check your local departmental policies on how these patients should be managed at this point. Some departments do not admit patients if they demonstrate they are able to swallow after aspiration. If in doubt, admit the patient and follow the general management principles above.

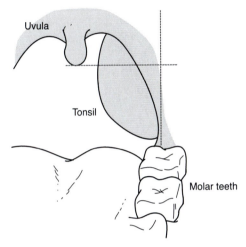

Point of aspiration is a crossing of a line drawn laterally from the inferior pole of the uvula to a line drawn superiorly from the molar teeth.

FIGURE 4.2 How to drain a quinsy.

Deep neck space infection/parapharyngeal abscess
If the patient has an associated diffuse swelling of the neck, then the infection may have spread into the deep neck spaces (parapharyngeal abscess). Discuss with your senior colleague as the patient may require a CT scan of the neck +/– surgery to drain the abscess.

Post-tonsillectomy haemorrhage

This can be very scary if you're new to this. The sight of blood pouring from someone's mouth is something you might only expect to see in horror films. However, it is a well-known complication of tonsillectomy, with around 4% returning to hospital and 1% requiring a return to the operating theatre. Mortality from post-tonsillectomy haemorrhage does happen so do not underestimate it, even if it seems like minor oozing only as this may herald a bigger bleed to come.

Post-tonsillectomy bleeding is divided into primary and secondary bleeds. Primary bleeding occurs within the first 24 hours of surgery and usually requires a return to theatre. Secondary bleeding can occur up to 14 days post-operatively and infection is thought to have a role. Treatment depends on severity, with a small number requiring return to theatre and the rest being successfully managed conservatively.

Preparation

Be prepared. A patient with active post-tonsillectomy haemorrhage may be spitting and coughing blood all around the emergency department. You must have adequate eye protection, gloves and an apron. Use a good headlight and a tongue depressor to get a decent view. Get a good assistant to give you a hand.

Initial management

Apply an ABC approach. A patient who is able to talk normally or a child who is crying demonstrates a satisfactory airway. A patient who is choking or struggling to breathe may have a clot in the airway that requires clearing. If there is a clot in the throat, try to clear it with a Yankauer sucker or a Magill's forceps. A patient with hypovolaemic shock will require appropriate fluid resuscitation and may require a blood transfusion. All patients should have IV access established and blood should be sampled for testing including FBC, U&E and clotting screen as a minimum. If you are not confident with children, ask the paediatricians for help. Patients should have a group and save if blood loss is minimal and the patient is stable, or a cross-match if a blood transfusion is needed. If the patient needs to go to theatre, appropriate resuscitation should be instigated whilst the patient is waiting to be transferred.

If there is active bleeding . . .

Adults and older children are asked to gargle hydrogen peroxide solution mixed as 1 part to 5 parts water for as long as is comfortable. They should spit it out into a bowl and must not swallow it! Reassess: If the bleeding has not stopped, try to identify the bleeding area in the tonsil fossa. If you can see it, roll up some cotton gauze soaked in 1:1000 adrenaline and hold it with a Magill's forceps. Press the gauze against the bleeding point continuously for as long as it is tolerable. The pressure and vasoconstriction may help control the bleeding. You can try cauterising the bleeding point with a silver nitrate stick. If bleeding persists, the patient needs to go to theatre. Inform your seniors, the anaesthetic team and theatres.

Young children need to go to theatre as soon as possible. They have small circulating volumes and observations only deteriorate when they have lost a significant amount of blood. Young children will swallow a lot of the blood, so you cannot assess blood loss very well. Call your seniors, the on-call anaesthetist and a paediatrician to help you.

If there is no active bleeding . . .

If there has been a small bleed that has resolved spontaneously, it is our view that these patients should also be admitted for observation and conservative management. This may be a herald bleed that precedes more significant haemorrhage.

Conservative management should be instigated, which includes, unless contraindicated, IV co-amoxiclav 1.2 g TDS and regular analgesia. In older children and adults, hydrogen peroxide gargles should be prescribed QDS (see above). The patient should be kept nil by mouth until senior review. IV fluids should be commenced for fluid replacement and maintenance if the patient is kept nil by mouth. If the patient rebleeds, they should be taken to theatre. Inform your senior, the anaesthetic team and theatre staff.

Nasal trauma

Britain is famous for sporting activities such as rugby and binge drinking. These pastimes may result in nasal trauma, sometimes in the form of fractured noses, particularly on a Friday or Saturday night. Some cases are attributable to elderly patients who have had falls. If you are asked to see these patients, do give thought to any underlying medical conditions that might have caused the fall. It is important to note that patients with nasal fractures may have other head injuries, and if you are called to assess these patients, assessment beyond the nose should also be undertaken. Ensure that ATLS guidelines have been followed and that primary survey and resuscitation has been undertaken prior to your assessment.

History

Timing and mechanism is important – make sure you document it well. A persistent bleed may indicate further intervention is needed (*see* 'Epistaxis', pp. 86–89). A clear discharge suggests CSF leak from a base of skull fracture. Nasal obstruction suggests septal deformity or haematoma. Visual disturbance (including double vision) may indicate orbital trauma or a 'blowout' fracture where the globe protrudes through a fracture in the floor of the orbit, causing diplopia on looking upwards. Dental malocclusion (a problem with bite) indicates a maxillary or mandibular fracture.

Examination

The nose should be examined from the front and above for any deviation, bruising or laceration. A subtle deviation will be more obvious from above. You should only be concerned with the nasal bones, as deviations in nasal septums can be corrected in the future. To the untrained, examination of the nose is difficult. First, lift the tip of the nose with your thumb to assess the anterior end of the internal nose. Using a headlight and Thudicum nasal speculum or an otoscope, look up both nostrils. Normally, you would find a clear airway with a straight septum. It is important to exclude a septal haematoma as if untreated this will lead to necrosis of the nasal septum and subsequent septal perforation and saddle deformity of the nose. Such an oversight may lead to an opportunity to rub shoulders with our medicolegal colleagues. A septal haematoma looks like a boggy swelling either side of the septum. If you suspect this, use a metal instrument such as a small forcep or probe, to press on the swelling – if it is boggy/soft and not painful, this may be a septal haematoma. If it is hard and painful when you press, it is probably the septal cartilage (medially) or the inferior turbinate (laterally).

Remember to assess for other facial fractures. Check for point tenderness over the maxillae and assess eye movements for signs of a blowout fracture. A facial X-ray can be requested for suspected facial fractures but never for a nasal fracture alone. It is important to look for any signs of skull base fractures such as CSF leak from the nose or ears, Battle's sign (bruising behind the ears) and raccoon eyes. If you are concerned, discuss with a senior colleague.

Management

It is most likely that you will encounter the patient a little while after their injury, during which time the nose becomes very swollen. It is not possible to make a definitive assessment until the swelling has resolved. You will need to wait 4–7 days for the inflammation to settle, so there is no point assessing them for manipulation prior to this. However, the nasal bones will set making manipulation difficult after

14 days. So this raises the challenge of assessing the nose for manipulation and performing the manipulation in this 7–10 day window. Arrange the appropriate follow-up for this. Many hospitals have ENT emergency clinics that these patients can be booked into. If you are unsure, take the patient's details and pass them on to the ENT team to sort out appropriate follow-up.

If a facial fracture, blowout fracture or fractured mandible is suspected, request appropriate X-rays and ask the maxillofacial team to review the patient.

If a septal haematoma is suspected, keep the patient nil by mouth and inform your senior colleague, as this patient will require urgent incision and drainage, insertion of a drain and nasal packing.

Pinna trauma

Pinna haematoma

If you watch or play rugby, you will have seen a cauliflower ear. These are lumpy ears that look like they have had a hard time. Pinna haematomas are normally caused by blunt trauma to the pinna, leading to bleeding between the perichondrium and the cartilage of the ear. The cartilage in the pinna gets its blood supply from the overlying perichondrium, so a haematoma disrupts this and if left will lead to necrosis of the cartilage and ultimately cauliflower ear.

These must be drained as an emergency by aspiration or by incision and drainage (the preferred option) usually under local anaesthetic. An incision is made over the haematoma and the clot is evacuated. The pocket is irrigated with normal saline. The wound is left open so that any further bleeding will drain out. To prevent recollection, the skin and cartilage of the pinna where the haematoma occurred should be 'sandwiched' between dental rolls (or silastic splints), which

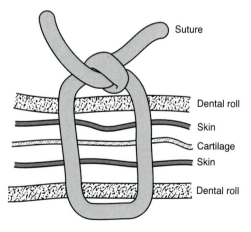

FIGURE 4.3 Pinna dressing.

are held in place using non-absorbable suture and a single stitch as shown in Figure 4.3 (it needs to be stable but not so tight as to cause necrosis!).

Pinna laceration

Lacerations through the pinna can look very intimidating to the untrained SHO who is asked to assess and repair them. Thankfully, they generally heal very well. Patients may present with anything from a small superficial cut that can be dealt with using tissue glue, to a partial or complete avulsion requiring significantly more to be done!

Applying first principles, if the pinna is pale and looks like it has no blood supply or has been completely avulsed from the head, you will need senior support and may need plastic surgeons to perform microvascular surgery to repair it. However, if there is some blood getting to the pinna, then there is a good chance it will recover well.

Depending on the size of the injury, either local infiltration or a pinna ring block will be needed to provide local anaesthesia to allow cleaning, irrigation with normal saline and suturing. Tetanus status should be checked and covered if needed. The key is to leave no exposed cartilage; if there has been skin loss, the surrounding skin can be undermined so it can be stretched over the cartilage, otherwise the exposed cartilage will have to be trimmed. Often it will be sufficient to close the skin with non-absorbable sutures, which will approximate the cartilage edges. If there is a doubt about this, then a couple of stitches with absorbable suture can be used to appose the cartilage edges prior to skin closure.

Local anaesthesia for the pinna

The pinna should be anaesthetised using lignocaine or equivalent (maximum dose 3 mg/kg), which will last up to an hour. Some argue that adrenaline should be avoided, but there is little evidence that doing so actually compromises the blood supply. Dental local anaesthetics are commonly used as they have a very fine needle and are easy to handle (2% lignocaine with 1:80000 adrenaline). Local injection alone can be used for small lacerations, but for larger injuries a pinna ring block can be performed, as demonstrated in Figure 4.4.

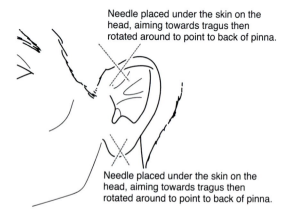

Needle placed under the skin on the head, aiming towards tragus then rotated around to point to back of pinna.

Needle placed under the skin on the head, aiming towards tragus then rotated around to point to back of pinna.

FIGURE 4.4 Pinna block.

After treating pinna trauma, a head bandage should be applied for a week (ideally use a non-adherent layer of dressing on the pinna, then cotton gauze and then crepe bandage). This should be stable but not so tight that it causes pain. Common practice is to prescribe prophylactic antibiotics (co-amoxiclav if there are no contraindications). The patient should be reviewed at 1 week when the dental rolls or sutures can be removed. Increasing pain may suggest haematoma and in this case the patient should be reviewed sooner.

Otitis externa

Otitus externa (OE) is inflammation of the external ear canal usually due to infection. It is a common ENT presentation featuring pain, discharge and oedema of the ear canal. The most common pathogen is *Pseudomonas aeruginosa*. Patients usually see their GPs, but some may present out of hours to hospital due to intolerable pain and ongoing symptoms. If a referral is made out of hours and the patient can wait, it is appropriate for the patient to be booked into the ENT emergency clinic within the next few days.

The examination should establish whether there is any surrounding cellulitis (pinna and face) and facial nerve weakness (it runs through the middle ear and the floor of the ear canal, so it can be affected by ear infections). Pull the pinna back or press the tragus gently to elicit tenderness, which is often present. A full cranial nerve examination should be undertaken. Use an otoscope to look in the ear canal, which can be straightened for a better view by pulling the pinna 'up and backwards' in adults and 'down and backwards' in children. OE is uncommon in children. If there is pus or debris in the ear canal you should clear it using microsuction (under the microscope using a Zoellner sucker). The availability of resources to do this out of hours will depend on your department, and you should have been trained, otherwise prescribe antibiotic drops and analgesia, and arrange for the patient to return for microsuction in the emergency clinic.

Following aural toilet, if the ear canal is patent and you can see the tympanic membrane, prescribe topical antibiotic ear drops and arrange for a review several days later. If the canal is very oedematous, and the tympanic membrane cannot be seen, ear drops will be ineffective because they will not penetrate the ear canal. This necessitates the insertion of an aural wick, which absorbs the drops and expands to open up the ear canal allowing the drops to work deep inside. Insertion is painful and is best done swiftly. Arrange for review in the ENT emergency clinic 48 hours later when the wick should be removed.

Topical antibiotic ear drops that include steroids are preferable (e.g. Sofradex or Gentisone HC®, 3 drops 3 times a day for 1 week). These are both aminoglycoside based, which are theoretically ototoxic, but the risk is justified by the need to treat the infection. Unless the tympanic membrane is perforated, these drops are not going to access the middle ear so this is not a concern. If there is a known perforation, ciprofloxacin eye drops are non-ototoxic and can be prescribed instead (though they are called eye drops they can be used in the ear also!). If you have a strong suspicion that the cause may be a fungal infection, you can use clotrimazole ear drops (fungal infections may occur where OE has been over-treated with topical antibiotics).

Oral antibiotics do not work for straightforward OE. They are only indicated if there is a spreading cellulitis (use co-amoxiclav), or furunculosis (infection of a hair follicle, use flucloxacillin). Furunculosis only occurs in the outer third of the ear canal, which is hair-bearing; abscesses might form that require lancing under local anaesthetic – arrange for senior review when appropriate.

Always be mindful of the possibility of malignant OE. Despite its name, it has nothing to do with cancer, but the name serves to underline how seriously it should be taken. It involves osteomyelitis of the temporal bone secondary to OE, which almost always occurs in elderly diabetics. It should always be considered in severe infections that are not responding to regular treatment where the pain seems disproportionately severe. The facial nerve can be affected so this must always be examined, as can other cranial nerves depending on which part of the skull base is involved. It is treated with at least 6 weeks of IV antibiotics as with any osteomyelitis. A full blood count, CRP and CT scan of the temporal bones should be requested.

Dermatological conditions, such as eczema, may be associated with OE, and are often preceded by itchy ear canals. These patients should be managed as already described, but may also benefit from a trial of early treatment during flare-ups with topical steroids (e.g. Betnovate scalp application 3 drops BD for 10 days).

All patients with OE must keep their ears dry to provide the best conditions for infection to resolve. Patients should be advised to take appropriate water precautions, such as using cotton wool soaked in petroleum jelly in the ear canal when taking a shower, and avoid baths and swimming, etc. This should continue for at least a week after the infection has cleared to allow full recovery.

A swab is only needed if the patient has had multiple courses of antibiotic drops, or if the pain is so severe that they require admission for analgesia. If the bugs are not sensitive to your chosen drops, they can be changed when the patient is reviewed depending on the sensitivities identified. The vast majority of these patients can be managed appropriately as outpatients. They only require admission if they have pinna or facial cellulitis, if they have facial nerve weakness suggesting malignant OE or if the pain is so severe that they require opiate analgesia.

Otitis media

Otitis media is inflammation of the middle ear, which is said to be acute or chronic depending on the duration (<3 weeks and >3 months respectively). Acute otitis media (AOM) is common in under-7s but can occur at any age. It often follows an upper respiratory tract infection (URTI). Impaired middle ear ventilation due to poor eustachian tube function causes an effusion, which may become infected causing earache. Examination may reveal a tympanic membrane that is bulging and hyperaemic. If the ear is discharging, there may also be a perforation and inflammation of the ear canal. Neurological assessment including cranial nerves should be undertaken to rule out focal neurology.

In uncomplicated cases of AOM, as with other URTIs, primary treatment is supportive. Patients should be given adequate analgesia and advised to maintain adequate hydration. Patients who are slow to recover may be prescribed antibiotics (amoxicillin or co-amoxiclav). If the patient suffers from three or more episodes within a 6-month period, a referral to ENT outpatients is recommended as they may benefit from grommet insertion. Most cases resolve spontaneously, which may involve rupture of the tympanic membrane allowing drainage of infected fluid and ventilation of the middle ear. The relief of pressure leads to a resolution of pain. Most tympanic membrane perforations will heal within a few weeks.

Chronic otitis media varies in presentation but may feature persistent tympanic membrane perforation (with or without discharge), granulation tissue or cholesteatoma. If there is active discharge, treat with topical antibiotic drops initially and arrange for ENT outpatient review if there are no complications.

Complications of otitis media can be considered as

intratemporal (within the temporal bone) and intracranial. Intratemporal complications include facial nerve palsy and acute mastoiditis. If the facial nerve is affected, myringotomy and grommet insertion may be necessary. This can wait until daytime. Acute mastoiditis describes the involvement of the mastoid bone with infection, as it is a direct continuation of the middle ear. This may result in a subperiosteal abscess, which presents as a hot, red, tender and fluctuant swelling behind the pinna, which may make the pinna protrude. Most cases of acute mastoiditis if treated early will respond to a period of IV antibiotics (co-amoxiclav if not contraindicated), but subperiosteal abscess will require surgical drainage. Inform your seniors if you suspect this.

Intracranial complications include meningitis, abscess (extradural, subdural or intracerebral) and lateral sinus thrombosis. Be suspicious if the patient is drowsy or there are neurological signs (focal signs, severe headache or evidence of meningism). If intracranial complications are suspected, discuss with your senior and request a CT scan of the brain with contrast in the first instance. Further tests may be indicated to guide treatment.

Otitis media with effusion is the technical term used to describe 'glue ear' in which the middle ear contains fluid that causes a conductive hearing loss. Following AOM, glue ear can persist for up to 3 months, beyond which it is considered to be chronic and less likely to resolve without intervention. This is not an emergency and can be seen in a routine ENT outpatient clinic.

Orbital cellulitis

This is an ENT emergency that can develop as a complication of acute rhinosinusitis. If left untreated it can lead to a permanent loss of vision. Infection can spread from the ethmoids through veins or the thin lamina papyracea bone that separates the nasal cavity from the orbit. In addition to examining the nose, you should check the pulse, blood pressure, temperature, eye appearance, eye movements and diplopia, colour vision, visual acuity, pupillary reflexes and palpate gently to elicit tenderness. Your senior and the ophthalmologists must assess these patients – if the vision is impaired this must happen immediately as the optic nerve is at risk! Urgent surgery may be needed.

Treatment consists of IV antibiotics, nasal steroids and nasal decongestants to treat the infection and decompress the sinus. An urgent CT scan of the sinuses with orbital sequences will be required. Surgery is required if there is abscess formation which can be either subperiosteal or within the orbit itself. If the patient does not need surgery, they should be reviewed regularly to identify deterioration. The infection may be termed pre-septal, which means that it is affecting the eyelid anterior to the 'orbital septum' (a membranous sheet that is the anterior limit of the orbit) and this will present with cellulitis and erythema of the eyelid and not eye or ENT symptoms. This will not require a CT scan or ENT treatment.

Other complications of acute rhinosinusitis include intracranial; cavernous sinus thrombosis, extradural abscess, subdural abscess, meningitis and intracerebral abscess and osseous; and osteomyelitis of the frontal bone (Pott's puffy tumour). If you suspect an intracranial complication, get a CT of the brain with contrast.

Further reading

Fokkens WJ, Lund VJ, Mullol J, *et al.* EPOS 2012: European position paper on rhinosinusitis and nasal polyps 2012. A summary for otorhinolaryngologists. *Rhinology.* 2012; **50**(1): 1–12.

Acute facial nerve palsy

Facial nerve (FN) palsy can be caused by upper motor neurone (UMN) and lower motor neurone (LMN) lesions. Forehead movement is intact in UMN lesions and affected in LMN lesions. Causes of UMN lesions include stroke, intracranial tumours and multiple sclerosis. Patients with UMN FN palsy should be referred to the medics.

The cause of LMN FN palsy should be established through history and examination. Investigations and treatment will be determined by the likely pathology. Examination should assess the ears, eyes, cranial nerves and parotid glands.

FN palsy is described using the House–Brackmann classification system:

Grade	Description of facial movement	Eyebrow lift?	Eye closure?	Smile
I	Normal	Yes	Complete	Normal
II	Slightly weak	Yes	Complete, min effort	Slight asymmetry
III	Obviously weak, not disfiguring	Yes/No	Complete, max effort	Obvious asymmetry
IV	Obviously weak, disfiguring	No	Incomplete	Obvious asymmetry
V	Barely perceptible	No	Incomplete	Minimal movement
VI	None at all	No	Incomplete	No movement

(Source: House JW, Brackmann DE. A facial nerve grading system. *Otolaryngol Head Neck Surg.* 1985 Apr; 93(2): 146–7.)

Grade IV implies that eye closure is incomplete, which requires certain precautions to prevent corneal injury. The affected eye should be treated with viscotears or hypromellose drops (2 drops QDS and PRN). Lacrilube ointment is used at night and the eyelids are taped closed horizontally with micropore tape (make sure the eyelashes are not pushed onto the cornea). Eyewear is recommended during the day, ideally an eye shield or spectacles with sides. An ophthalmology opinion should be sought if the eye becomes very sore and red.

Common causes of acute facial nerve palsy

Idiopathic (Bell's palsy)

Bell's palsy is thought to be secondary to herpes simplex infection of the FN and is a diagnosis of exclusion, so history and examination is focused on ruling out other causes. If the patient presents within 48 hours of onset, prescribe prednisolone 50 mg for 5 days as this may improve recovery. Antivirals are also commonly prescribed (acyclovir 200 mg for 10 days), but there is little evidence for this. Reassure the patient that over 70% will fully resolve within 2 months. Arrange follow-up at 6 weeks in outpatients with an audiogram on arrival.

Ramsay Hunt syndrome

Ramsay Hunt syndrome is secondary to reactivation of dormant varicella zoster virus in the FN ganglia (shingles of the facial nerve). It differs from Bell's palsy, as there are features additional to FN palsy: vesicles are seen in the concha of the external ear (sensation in this area is supplied by the FN) and it is painful. Following recovery these patients can have severe post-herpetic neuralgia, so it is important to treat them acutely with antivirals to reduce this (acyclovir 800 mg 5 times a day for 10 days). Also prescribe prednisolone 50 mg for 5 days. Arrange follow-up at 6 weeks in outpatients with an audiogram on arrival.

Other causes

Infective: acute otitis media, malignant otitis externa.
Traumatic: temporal bone fractures.
Iatrogenic: post-parotid and middle ear surgery.
Neoplastic: tumours along the course of facial nerve (brainstem, internal auditory meatus, middle ear, skull base or parotid).

Chapter 5

ORTHOPAEDICS

Benjamin Bradley and
Al-Amin Kassam

Assessment of radiographs

Remember the basics.
- ➲ **Name**
- ➲ **Date of exam**
- ➲ **Views**
- ➲ **Adequacy**
- ➲ **Body part**

Fracture line and fragments

Describe how many fragments there are. All fractures have at least two fragments. Simple fractures are two-part fractures and comminuted fractures describe any fracture that has more than two parts.

- ➲ Transverse – a fracture at a right angle to the long axis of the bone.
- ➲ Oblique fracture – a fracture that is diagonal to a bone's long axis. Only visible on one view.
- ➲ Spiral fracture – a fracture where at least one part of the bone has been twisted. Visible on two separate orthogonal views, usually an AP and lateral.

Fracture site

Fracture sites can be described in terms of parts of the bone:

- ➲ epiphysis
- ➲ metaphysis
- ➲ diaphysis.

They can also include specific parts of the bone, e.g. head, neck, spine, etc. Long bones are also often arbitrarily divided into proximal, middle and distal thirds.

Joint involvement

There are joints at either end of the bone and thus fractures can also be:

➲ intra-articular = extending into the joint
➲ extra-articular = *not* extending into the joint.

Intra-articular fractures normally require anatomical reduction (i.e. operative fixation) to restore function, whereas extra-articular fractures require only alignment of the bony fragments.

Deformity

Bones are three-dimensional structures and deformity can occur in any dimension. There are four key features to describe when discussing the deformity of a bone: apposition, angulation, rotation and bone length. Together they affect the alignment of the bone and constitute displacement.

Convention dictates that deformity is described in relation to the distal fragment

Apposition refers to the amount of bony contact evident at the fracture site. If a fragment has moved on another, then this is termed **translation**. Apposition is described as a percentage of the amount of contact. A fragment that has displaced by 100% can be described as 'off-ended'.

Angulation (measured in degrees) refers to the amount of divergence from the normal axis of the bone. This can happen in any plane (think three dimensions), so two views are really important. One view is always one view too few.

Rotation is simple to understand but harder to assess on two-dimensional images. Discrepancies in diameter of bone above and below or a difference in cortical thickness above and below is suspicious of rotation. An easier way of assessing fracture rotation is to include the joints above and below the fracture on the X-ray.

Shortening of the bone can be caused by a fracture. This can be difficult to assess when looking at views taken only at the fracture site.

Basic principles of management

Once the fracture has been described further management needs to be considered. Orthopaedics can be simplified to the three Rs:

- ⮑ Reduce
- ⮑ Retain
- ⮑ Rehabilitate

Reduction is important if deformity is present. Retention of a fracture position whether after reduction or not can be non-operative (sometimes called conservative) or operative.

Surgical management can be further subdivided into internal or external fixation. Internal fixation can be achieved by a variety of methods and is further subclassified into intra- or extramedullary fixation.

Open fractures

An open fracture is any fracture in which the broken bone has penetrated the skin. This section is aimed at giving you a system to provide first aid treatment to any open fracture. Each injury will require specific definitive treatment.

Assessment

> **You need to assess the:**
> - size of the wound
> - extent of tissue damage/loss – skin, muscle periosteum
> - associated vascular and/or nerve injury
> - degree of contamination.

Open fractures often occur as a result of high energy trauma. Therefore the patient should initially be assessed and resuscitated according to ATLS principles.

Any wound associated with an underlying fracture should be considered to be an open fracture. Once the patient has been stabilised then the open fracture can be assessed, usually as part of the secondary survey.

Gustilo and Anderson classification

Grade I: wound <1 cm, no contamination, minimal muscle damage and simple fracture pattern. This is usually an inside to outside type injury.

Grade II: wound >1 cm. There can be moderate levels of soft tissue injury, contamination and comminution.

Grade III: any open fracture with high levels of contamination, extensive soft tissue injury or neurovascular injury:

- IIIa: extensive soft tissue laceration with adequate bone coverage
- IIIb: extensive soft tissue injury with periosteal stripping and exposed bone
- IIIc: associated vascular injury.

Classification

It is useful to grade the open fracture at the initial assessment, as this guides further management of the injury.

The Gustilo and Anderson classification system is commonly used. This was originally described for the intraoperative assessment of open fractures but is also useful for the initial assessment.

Management

> **First aid management of open fractures**
> - Remove gross contamination.
> - Reduce exposed bone where possible.
> - Photograph injury.
> - Cover wound with sterile gauze soaked either in saline or Betadine.
> - IV antibiotics according to local policy.
> - Splint fracture.

For any open fracture, the first aid management is the same and needs to be done immediately. You need to keep the patient nil by mouth, arrange appropriate X-rays and inform your registrar.

The wound needs exploration, washout and debridement with appropriate skeletal stabilisation in theatre as soon as possible. Recent guidelines have allowed a slight relaxation on the timing of surgery depending on the nature of the injury. Essentially the surgery needs to be performed at an appropriate time, by an appropriate surgeon, with appropriate theatre staff and the correct kit available. For a Gustilo and Anderson grade I open fracture, this may be the next trauma list within 12–24 hours. However, for more extensive injuries surgery needs to be performed as an emergency procedure within 6 hours of injury.

Acute compartment syndrome

Acute compartment syndrome is one of the true orthopaedic emergencies. This is a limb-threatening condition and delayed or missed diagnosis will have disastrous consequences. It is therefore important that you have a very high index of suspicion. Any patient with suspected compartment syndrome must be seen as a priority and definitely warrants immediate senior opinion.

Basic science

For trauma-meeting purposes this definition is a good one:

> 'elevation of the interstitial pressure in a closed osseofascial compartment that results in microvascular compromise'.

An insult to normal local tissue homeostasis within the compartment results in swelling and an increased tissue pressure due to the relative inelastic nature of the osseofascial compartment. This compromises venous drainage, which further raises the tissue pressure within the compartment. The compartment pressure continues to increase, resulting in the capillary perfusion pressure being exceeded, which leads to oxygen deprivation and ultimately tissue necrosis.

Causes

The most common cause of acute compartment syndrome is fracture of the bone within that compartment. However, there are a number of other causes and it is really important that you are aware of these so you can reduce the chance of missing a compartment syndrome.

> **Causes of acute compartment syndrome:**
> - fractures
> - soft tissue trauma
> - arterial injury
> - limb compression during altered consciousness – remember post-operative patients who have had long tourniquet times
> - burns
> - casts.

It is important to remember that external compression on a limb from a cast can cause an acute compartment pressure. If this is recognised early, then splitting and/or removing the cast can restore normal haemodynamics to the compartment before any irreversible damage occurs.

Sites

The most common site for an acute compartment syndrome is the **lower leg**, usually as a result of a **diaphyseal tibial fracture**. Less commonly, an acute compartment syndrome can occur in the forearm, thigh, hand or foot.

If you are doing well in the morning trauma meeting, you may be asked about the compartments of the lower leg. There are four compartments in the lower leg: anterior, deep posterior, superficial posterior and peroneal. Acute compartment syndrome most commonly occurs in the anterior compartment followed by the deep posterior.

If you are really flying, then the boss may ask you to draw an anatomical cross-section of the mid-tibia region.

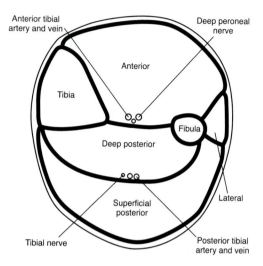

FIGURE 5.1 Compartments of the lower leg.

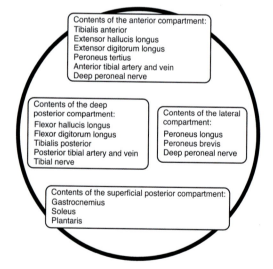

Contents of the anterior compartment:
Tibialis anterior
Extensor hallucis longus
Extensor digitorum longus
Peroneus tertius
Anterior tibial artery and vein
Deep peroneal nerve

Contents of the deep posterior compartment:
Flexor hallucis longus
Flexor digitorum longus
Tibialis posterior
Posterior tibial artery and vein
Tibial nerve

Contents of the lateral compartment:
Peroneus longus
Peroneus brevis
Deep peroneal nerve

Contents of the superficial posterior compartment:
Gastrocnemius
Soleus
Plantaris

FIGURE 5.2 Compartments of the lower leg.

Diagnosis

Acute compartment syndrome usually occurs within the first 24 hours of injury and is rare beyond 48 hours. The most important presenting feature is **pain**. Compartment syndrome must be considered whenever the pain is out of proportion with the nature of the injury.

The key examination finding is **pain on passive stretch** of the muscles in the affected compartment. It is important that you remember your anatomy in order to properly assess this. For example, the most commonly affected compartment is the anterior compartment of the lower leg. This compartment contains tibialis anterior and the long toe extensors; you therefore have to flex the toes to stretch this compartment.

The other crucial examination finding is a **tense, tender compartment**. The features of an acute compartment syndrome are classically described as the 'five Ps': pain, paraesthesia, pallor, paralysis and pulselessness. Other than pain, these are late features and if present represent a high risk of irreversible tissue ischaemia. You need to recognise compartment syndrome before it reaches this point.

Management plan

This is an emergency and you need to act now. If the patient has a cast applied, then open it immediately. You must contact the orthopaedic registrar now.

If the clinical picture is not clear, you may be asked to perform compartment pressure monitoring. Use of compartment pressure monitors is important and SHOs need to be aware of their existence. Each orthopaedic department will have access to a hand-held compartment pressure monitor. The instructions for the monitor will be available with the kit. Essentially, you need to insert the needle into the compartment and the monitor will automatically record the pressure.

If the compartment pressure exceeds **30 mmHg**, this is highly indicative of compartment syndrome. A compartment pressure within 30 mmHg of the diastolic blood pressure is also used to indicate a compartment pressure, as this allows for permissive hypotension resuscitation.

If a compartment syndrome is suspected, **emergency fasciotomies** must be performed. The anaesthetists and theatre staff must be informed and the patient will need to be marked and consented. A two-incision technique should be used to decompress all four compartments. The entire length of each compartment must be decompressed. There is no place for small incisions when performing emergency fasciotomies. The **anterolateral incision** accesses the anterior compartment. It should extend the entire length of the lower leg, and is placed anterior to the fibula over

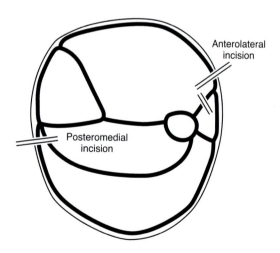

FIGURE 5.3 Incisions for lower leg fasciotomy.

the anterior compartment. The lateral compartment is also accessed through this incision. The **posteromedial incision** should be just posterior to the medial border of the tibia and again extend the entire length of the lower leg. The incision is through the superficial compartment and into the deep posterior compartment.

Spines

History

The mechanism and extent of injury can be vital in predicting injuries not seen on examination and basic radiographs. Document the exact time, context and mechanism of injury. Full and thorough documentation of history and examination is imperative in spinal assessment, as symptom deterioration or improvement is often used in significant management decisions and allows good handover to senior colleagues and spinal surgeons.

Examination

Undertake and document a full spinal and neurological assessment and logrolling if spine not cleared post-trauma.

Assess for:

- ◐ tenderness
- ◐ bruising
- ◐ changes in normal alignment (e.g. steps, gaps, etc.).

	Sensation	Power		Sensation	Power
C5	Badge area over deltoid	Elbow flexion	L2	Mid thigh anteriorly	Hip flexion
C6	Thumb	Wrist extension	L3	Patella	Knee extension
C7	Middle finger	Elbow extension	L4	Medial calf	Ankle dorsiflexion
C8	Little finger	Finger flexion	L5	Big toe	Big toe extension
T1	Medial aspect elbow	Little finger abduction	S1	Heel	Ankle plantar flexion

A full neurological examination includes tone, sensation, power and reflexes (upper limb: biceps, triceps and supinator; lower limb: patella, ankle and plantars). Markers at which to assess sensation and power are listed in the table above.

Digital rectal examination should be performed – document perianal sensation and anal tone.

Cervical spine clearance

Most can be cleared clinically by careful examination, *but* for major trauma, altered mental status, neurological deficit or with distracting injuries (e.g. long bone fractures, rib fracture, abdominal injuries), clinical examination and radiological clearance (with radiographs and/or CT) must be undertaken together.

If there is any doubt involved, the cervical spine immobilisation should be continued until definitive proof of no injury can be shown.

If no abnormality is found on spinal or neurological examination, remove the immobilisation and allow gentle flexion, extension and rotation of the neck. If this continues to be pain-free, then clearance is achieved. If any pain occurs, replace the immobilisation.

Cervical spine radiographic clearance (need a radiograph)

SHOs covering Trauma and Orthopaedics should have a working knowledge of clearing a cervical spine using radiographs. Radiographs obtained are the lateral view, AP and open-mouth peg view. The easiest way to remember is using ABCD.

Adequacy – does the radiograph show from the base of the skull to the C7/T1 junction?

Alignment – are the anterior, posterior, spinolaminar lines smooth and in continuity?
– Is the peg view symmetrical, i.e. sitting centrally between the lateral masses?

Bones – are there any obvious fractures on any view?

'**C**'oft tissues – is there significant soft tissue swelling anteriorly to the vertebral bodies. The general rule is the soft tissue shadow in front of the vertebral body should be no more than 50% of the width of the body for the C2–C4 vertebrae and no more than 100% of the width of the vertebral bodies for the C5–C7 vertebrae.

Dislocation – on the AP view the facet joints should all line up and lie on top of each other like tiles.

Always remember if there is any doubt radiological assessment with CT and or MRI should be considered along with senior review.

Basic management of spinal fractures

Spinal fractures can be treated with the same principles as fractures of other bones. Fractures need to be immobilised (i.e. cervical collar, bed rest) until the fracture has been shown to be stable/unstable. If there is any neurological compromise, urgent senior advice should be sought.

Stable fractures can normally be managed non-operatively with unstable fractures needing surgical intervention. Mechanical spinal stability is explained using Denis's three-column model. The spine is formed of three columns: anterior, middle and posterior columns.

Anterior column	Middle column	Posterior column
Anterior half vertebral body	Posterior half of vertebral body	Facet joints including facet joint capsule
Anterior half of intervertebral disc	Posterior half of intervertebral disc	Posterior ligamentous complex (interspinal ligaments, ligamentum flavum)
Anterior longitudinal ligament (ALL)	Posterior longitudinal ligament (PLL)	Laminae and pedicles

(Source: Denis F. The three column spine and its significance in the classification of acute thoracolumbar spinal injuries. *Spine* (Phila PA 1976). 1983 Nov–Dec; **8**(8): 817–31.)

Mechanical stability post injury can be assessed after assessment of the patient's pain, deformity and neurological status along with their mechanism of injury and the injury to the three columns of the spine. In conjunction, a decision can be made of spinal stability and treatment required. This should be made by a senior clinician or spinal surgeon. If there is any doubt, keep the patient immobilised in a cervical spine collar for cervical spine fractures on bed rest with strict logrolling for other fractures.

Specific management

Transverse process fractures

Transverse process fractures are generally stable if not associated with other bony or soft tissue spinal injury. Injury of more than four transverse processes should raise suspicions of other spinal injury (especially soft tissues) and needs further imaging.

Wedge compression fractures

Wedge compression fractures are generally stable and rarely involve neurological compromise. The anterior column alone is involved. Treatment involves analgesia and spinal bracing if pain is uncontrolled. Compression of >50% of the vertebral body height or multiple adjacent compression fractures can be considered potentially unstable. Care needs to be taken to exclude burst fractures when assessing wedge compression fractures.

Burst fractures

Burst fractures are unstable. Both anterior and posterior walls of the vertebral bodies are fractured. Fracture of the posterior body can involve retropulsion of bone into the spinal canal and can lead to neurological compromise. Further imaging (CT/MRI) and discussion with senior colleagues or spinal surgeons is needed.

Spinal cord injury

Trauma can lead to spinal cord injury and the injury (whether complete or incomplete) needs to be communicated when discussing the patient with colleagues and spinal surgeons.

Complete spinal cord injury

There will be total motor and sensory loss distal to the spinal injury level.

Incomplete spinal cord injury

If incomplete, some motor or sensory function will be present distal to the spinal injury level.

- ➲ Brown-Séquard syndrome: this is caused by hemisection of the cord due to pedicle fracture or penetrating injury. Symptoms include motor weakness of the side of the lesion and contralateral loss of pain and temperature sensation. There is good prognosis for recovery.
- ➲ Anterior cord syndrome: this is usually caused by a

hyperflexion injury in which there is compression of the anterior spinal artery and spinal cord. Symptoms include complete loss of motor and sensory function distal to the spinal level and prognosis is poor.

- ➲ Central cord syndrome: this is the most common type of incomplete spinal cord injury. The centrally located tracts for arm function are affected more than the peripherally located leg tracts, so patients present with loss of motor and sensory function in the arms with often well-preserved leg function. It usually occurs as a result of hyperextension injury, usually in an older person with pre-existing spinal stenosis.

Cauda equina syndrome

Cauda equina syndrome is most commonly caused by a large midline intervertebral disc prolapse causing nerve root compression. Rarer causes include infection, trauma, spinal stenosis and post-surgery or spinal anaesthetic (e.g. epidural haematoma).

Presentation is with severe lower back pain (often significantly worse than their normal back pain) and faecal or urinary incontinence or retention. Symptoms are often incomplete. Assessment must include digital rectal examination to assess perianal sensation and anal sphincter tone.

Cauda equina is a surgical emergency and, if suspicious, an urgent MRI is needed followed by urgent surgical decompression of the nerve roots.

Radiculopathy

Radicular symptoms arise from compression of the nerve roots and mainly present as radiating pain in the distribution of the nerve roots. Most commonly this presents as buttock and leg pain, although it can affect the arms (brachalgia).

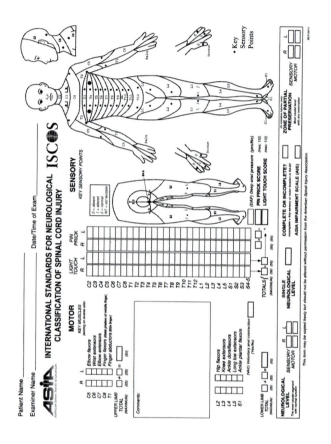

FIGURE 5.4 ASIA chart. Reprinted from American Spinal Injury Association. *International Standards for Neurological Classification of Spinal Cord Injury*, revised 2011. Atlanta, GA: ASIA; 2011.

Muscle Function Grading

0 = total paralysis

1 = palpable or visible contraction

2 = active movement, full range of motion (ROM) with gravity eliminated

3 = active movement, full ROM against gravity

4 = active movement, full ROM against gravity and moderate resistance in a muscle specific position.

5 = (normal) active movement, full ROM against gravity and full resistance in a muscle specific position expected from an otherwise unimpaired person.

5* = (normal) active movement, full ROM against gravity and sufficient resistance to be considered normal if identified inhibiting factors (i.e. pain, disuse) were not present.

NT= not testable (i.e. due to immobilization, severe pain such that the patient cannot be graded, amputation of limb, or contracture of >50% of the range of motion).

ASIA Impairment (AIS) Scale

☐ **A = Complete.** No sensory or motor function is preserved in the sacral segments S4-S5.

☐ **B = Sensory Incomplete.** Sensory but not motor function is preserved below the neurological level and includes the sacral segments S4-S5 (light touch, pin prick at S4-S5: or deep anal pressure (DAP)), AND no motor function is preserved more than three levels below the motor level on either side of the body.

☐ **C = Motor Incomplete.** Motor function is preserved below the neurological level**, and more than half of key muscle functions below the single neurological level of injury (NLI) have a muscle grade less than 3 (Grades 0-2).

☐ **D = Motor Incomplete.** Motor function is preserved below the neurological level**, and _at least half (half or more) of key muscle functions_ below the NLI have a muscle grade ≥ 3.

☐ **E = Normal.** If sensation and motor function as tested with the ISNCSCI are graded as normal in all segments, and the patient had prior deficits, then the AIS grade is E. Someone without an initial SCI does not receive an AIS grade.

**For an individual to receive a grade of C or D, i.e. motor incomplete status, they must have either (1) voluntary anal sphincter contraction or (2) sacral sensory sparing with sparing of motor function more than three levels below the motor level for that side of the body. The Standards at this time allows even non-key muscle function more than 3 levels below the motor level to be used in determining motor incomplete status (AIS B versus C).

NOTE: When assessing the extent of motor sparing below the level for distinguishing between AIS B and C, the _motor level_ on each side is used, whereas to differentiate between AIS C and D (based on proportion of key muscle functions with strength grade 3 or greater) the _single neurological level_ is used.

Steps in Classification

The following order is recommended in determining the classification of individuals with SCI.

1. Determine sensory levels for right and left sides.

2. Determine motor levels for right and left sides.
   Note: in regions where there is no myotome to test, the motor level is presumed to be the same as the sensory level, if testable motor function above that level is also normal.

3. Determine the single neurological level.
   This is the lowest segment where motor and sensory function is normal on both sides, and is the most cephalad of the sensory and motor levels determined in steps 1 and 2.

4. Determine whether the injury is Complete or Incomplete.
   (i.e. absence or presence of sacral sparing)
   If voluntary anal contraction = **No** AND all S4-5 sensory scores = **0** AND deep anal pressure = **No**, then injury is COMPLETE. Otherwise, injury is incomplete.

5. Determine ASIA Impairment Scale (AIS) Grade:
   If YES, AIS=A and can record ZPP (lowest dermatome or myotome on each side with some preservation)

   Is injury Complete?
   ↓ NO

   Is injury motor Incomplete? → If NO, AIS=B
   (Yes=voluntary anal contraction OR motor function more than three levels below the motor level on a given side, if the patient has sensory incomplete classification)
   ↓ YES

   Are at least half of the key muscles below the single neurological level graded 3 or better?

   NO ↓ ↓ YES

   AIS=C   AIS=D

   If sensation and motor function is normal in all segments, AIS=E
   Note: AIS E is used in follow-up testing when an individual with a documented SCI has recovered normal function. If at initial testing no deficits are found, the individual is neurologically intact; the ASIA Impairment Scale does not apply.

Neurological signs are rare although lower motor neurone signs may be present. Isolated radicular pain requires analgesia with specialist physiotherapy. Surgery is only indicated if prolonged non-operative treatment has failed or if any signs of cauda equina compression are present.

Discitis

This is infection centred around the intervertebral disc and presents as severe lower back pain and is often associated with radicular nerve root pain and signs of infection (pyrexia, systemic malaise, fevers, etc.).

A full septic screen should be performed and other causes of sepsis excluded. Three sets of blood cultures should be taken to obtain bacteriological diagnosis prior to commencing antibiotics (unless the patient is systemically unwell in which case antibiotics can be started empirically). This may require disc biopsy if blood cultures are negative.

Definitive diagnosis is made with MRI scan. If the infection is confined to the disc space, treatment is with a prolonged course of intravenous and oral antibiotics. Surgery may be needed to drain collections.

Pelvic fractures

Pelvic fractures are life-threatening injuries. The mechanism is usually high-energy trauma and patients should present as a trauma call. Pelvic injury is assessed for in the C part of the ATLS primary survey. If your registrar is not part of the trauma team, then you should contact them immediately when a pelvic injury is suspected.

Associated injuries

The immediate life-threatening complication of pelvic fractures is blood loss. There are three possible sources of blood loss:

- ○ pelvic venous plexus
- ○ pelvic arterial injury
- ○ fractured bone ends.

Injury to the venous plexus, which lies on the anterior surface of the sacrum, is the most common source of blood loss with pelvic fractures. There is also a high association with injury to intraperitoneal and retroperitoneal visceral structures (urethra, bladder, rectum and vagina). If there are associated injuries to the rectum or vagina, these should be considered to be open fractures.

Assessment

This should occur within the ATLS primary survey. Initially you need assessment of the haemodynamic status of the patient, with basic resuscitation. Severe pelvic fractures may be demonstrated by abnormal leg positions, such as externally rotated legs or leg length discrepancy.

You should also inspect the pelvis for external signs of internal injury:

- ○ perineal and flank bruising indicating haemorrhage

- ⭢ blood at urethral meatus indicating urethral injury
- ⭢ perineal laceration
- ⭢ lacerations/blood on PR and PV examinations
- ⭢ high-riding prostate on PR.

X-ray interpretation

You should inspect the AP pelvis radiograph for signs of:

- ◐ anterior injuries – widening of the pubic symphysis, pubic rami fractures
- ◐ posterior injuries – widening of the sacro-iliac joints, sacral fractures, L5 transverse process fractures
- ◐ iliac fractures.

If a pelvic fracture is suspected, then a pelvic binder should be applied. There are many different devices available that all essentially function in the same way. The most important thing is to ensure that you apply the binder in the correct position – the binder should be centred on the greater trochanters of the hips; this will look much lower than expected. If there is no evidence of a urethral injury, then you should insert a urinary catheter in order to monitor volaemic status.

Once the primary survey is complete, a trauma series of radiographs will be performed. An AP pelvis view will be performed as part of this trauma series. If there is clinical evidence and/or radiographic features of a pelvic fracture, then the patient should have a CT scan if they are stable enough.

Classification

Young and Burgess is the most commonly used classification system. You should know the basics of this very useful system. It is based on the mechanism of injury and indicates possible associated injuries.

Lateral compression (LC) injuries

A laterally applied force compresses that side of the pelvis inwards. There is a high risk of associated injury to visceral structures.

LC-I: sacral impaction on the side of impact. There may be associated undisplaced pubic rami fractures on that side. Stable injury with low incidence of associated injuries.

LC-II: posterior iliac wing fracture with pubic rami fracture. The hemipelvis is forced inwards providing a high risk of visceral damage and possible arterial injury.

LC-III: as the impacted side is forced inward there is opening of the contralateral hemipelvis.

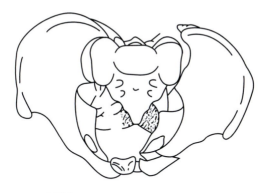

FIGURE 5.5 LC-III injury.

AP compression injuries

These result from an AP compressive force which forces the two hemipelvises apart. There is always injury to the anterior pelvis but the key to assessing the severity is to identify injury to the posterior structures.

These injuries progress from minimal opening of the anterior pelvis through to full 'open book' injuries in which the hemipelvises are significantly externally rotated. There is a high incidence of vascular injury and haemodynamic instability with opening of the pelvis.

- ⊃ APC-I: slight widening of pubic symphysis or relatively undisplaced pubic rami fractures. Anterior SI joint ligaments are stretched but intact.
- ⊃ APC-II: Anterior pelvic injury with disruption of the anterior SI joint ligaments but intact posterior SI joint ligaments.
- ⊃ APC-III: anterior pelvic injury with complete disruption and opening of SI joints.

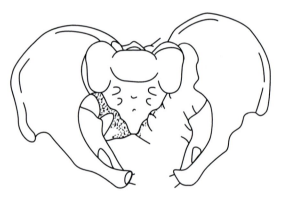

FIGURE 5.6 APC-II injury.

Vertical shear injuries

These often result from falls. A vertical or longitudinally applied force is applied which forces one hemipelvis upwards. There is usually complete disruption of the symphysis, sacrotuberous, sacrospinous and sacroiliac ligaments. There is a high incidence of associated neurological and vascular injuries.

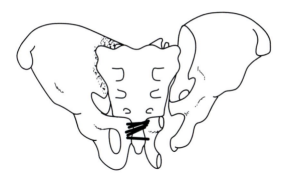

FIGURE 5.7 Vertical shear.

Combined mechanism

This is a combination of mechanisms of injuries and has unpredictable injury patterns.

Definitive treatment

If you can assess pelvic fractures and institute appropriate immediate management then you will be doing well and definitive treatment will be down to your seniors.

Essentially unstable pelvises need to be reduced and stabilised. A patient who is haemodynamically unstable will need emergent treatment. Bleeding from the venous sacral plexus will need to be packed at formal open operation. Arterial bleeding may respond to embolisation.

Pelvic binders can be left in place for about 12 hours, any longer risks pressure areas and tissue necrosis. If it is not possible to perform open reduction internal fixation at this stage, then a pelvic external fixator should be applied.

Hip fractures

Admitting hip fractures will be the bread and butter of your work as an orthopaedic SHO. You will usually see at least one per shift and your main role is to ensure that the patient is medically stable.

Anatomy

It is crucial that you are able to distinguish between intracapsular and extracapsular hip fractures.

The capsule encloses the femoral head and hip joint. It attaches anteriorly at the intertrochanteric line and posteriorly about 1 cm proximal to the intertrochanteric line.

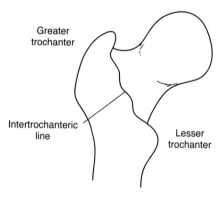

Greater trochanter

Intertrochanteric line

Lesser trochanter

FIGURE 5.8 Attachments of the hip capsule.

The femoral head has a predominantly retrograde blood supply. The profunda femoris artery supplies an anastomotic ring between the medial and lateral circumflex femoral arteries at the base of the hip capsule. Retinacular arteries arise from this anastomotic ring and pass up the femoral neck to supply the head. Other less significant sources of blood to the femoral head are the diaphyseal vessels and the artery in the ligamentum teres (negligible after childhood). The blood supply to the femoral head is compromised with displaced intracapsular fractures. The important retinacular blood vessels are stretched and probably torn.

Intracapsular hip fractures

These fractures occur proximal to the intertrochanteric line. They can be displaced or undisplaced.

Garden's classification is most commonly used to describe intracapsular hip fractures. This classification system is based on the AP X-rays only.

Garden's classification:

- ◘ I and II – undisplaced fractures (blood supply likely intact)
- ◘ III and IV – displaced fractures (blood supply likely compromised).

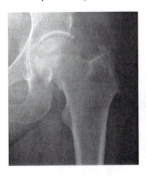 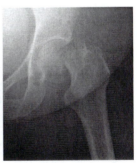

FIGURE 5.9 (a) Undisplaced and (b) displaced IC fracture.

Extracapsular hip fractures

These fractures occur distal to the intertrochanteric line. The retinacular blood vessels that pass proximally in the hip capsule are undamaged. The blood supply to the femoral head is not compromised in extracapsular fractures.

Intertrochanteric fractures occur between the greater and lesser trochanters in the metaphyseal area of bone.

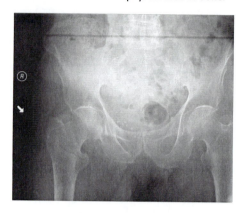

FIGURE 5.10 Intertrochanteric fracture.

Subtrochanteric fractures occur below the level of the trochanters.

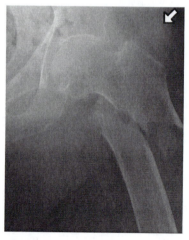

FIGURE 5.11 Subtrochanteric fracture.

Patient assessment

You will be referred a patient by the A&E doctor as 'a NOF'. Unfortunately, the referral is often based on an X-ray alone and it will be your job to do a full patient assessment and start initial management.

A patient under 65 years with a displaced intracapsular hip fracture is an orthopaedic emergency. The blood supply to the femoral head is threatened. The fracture needs to be reduced and fixed as soon as possible to try and restore blood supply. You will need to inform your registrar of this patient immediately and prepare them for theatre.

The vast majority of patients who sustain a hip fracture are old people who sustain a low-energy fall. Your main role in the initial assessment of these patients is to assess why they fell and ensure that they are medically stable.

History can be difficult, especially if the patient is demented. You need to get as much information as possible, using relatives and carers where needed. You need to distinguish between medical and mechanical falls. If you suspect a medical cause, contact the medical team for advice. You also need to be aware of the possibility of pathological fractures, particularly where there is minimal trauma. You should ask about preceding hip/leg pain and go through the systemic features of malignancy. A full social history including exercise tolerance and walking ability is important as it helps to guide management.

Examination

The leg is often short and externally rotated due to the unopposed action of the powerful hip flexors that remain inserted around the lesser trochanter. You need to document the neurovascular status and skin condition.

A full systemic examination is needed in order to identify

possible causes for the fall and assess fitness for anaesthesia. If a pathological fracture is suspected then PR and breast examination will be additionally indicated.

Investigations

ECG, chest X-ray and pre-operative bloods are the basic investigations required in addition to the AP pelvis and lateral hip radiograph.

Initial management

Ilio-fascial block

This can be performed for patients with a neck of femur fracture and is safer and offers better pain relief compared to an isolated femoral nerve block. A medium-acting local anaesthetic should be utilised (e.g. bupivicaine 0.5%; up to 2.5 mg/kg body weight can be used, but normally 20 mL of 0.5% can be safely used in most adult patients).

A line should be drawn between the anterior superior iliac spine (ASIS) and the pubic symphysis. The junction between the middle third and the lateral third should be identified and injection of the local anaesthetic should be given 2 cm distal to this point. The needle should be inserted through two fascial layers (tensor fascia lata and fascia iliaca), identified by the loss of resistance on penetrating each layer. Once this double loss of resistance is felt, the local anaesthetic can be injected safely.

The patient will require adequate analgesia usually in the form of paracetamol, codeine/tramadol and oramorph. Some units will use a iliac fascia block for additional pain relief.

These patients are often dry and IV fluids should be given to rehydrate them. Be careful not to overload the patient though.

The patient should be given some form of low-molecular-weight heparin as your department dictates and prepared for the next available trauma list. If a patient is anticoagulated, this is likely to need to be reversed – the exact way to reverse will depend on the reason for the anticoagulation. Medical input is often helpful.

Definitive treatment

The mortality of untreated hip fractures is approaching 100%. It is therefore important that these fractures are treated operatively in order to prevent immobility and the inevitable consequences of this. Even with operative treatment of these fractures the mortality rates are still incredibly high. One-month mortality rates are around 33%, with mortality rates of 35% at 1 year. Current guidelines state that patients should undergo operative treatment within the first 24 hours of injury in order to reduce the risk of complications.

Displaced intracapsular hip fracture in elderly patients

The blood supply to the femoral head has been destroyed and therefore these fractures will not unite. The femoral head is therefore removed and a form of arthroplasty is performed.

In low-demand, frail patients a hemiarthroplasty is usually performed. In higher-demand, fitter patients a total hip replacement is often considered.

Undisplaced intracapsular fracture

The blood supply has probably not been disturbed and therefore it is possible to fix these fractures. Cannulated screws or a two-hole dynamic hip screw (DHS) are usually used to internally fix the fracture. A period of protected weight bearing is required post-operatively and in old, frail patients who may also be demented this is often not possible. In these patients a one-stop single procedure in the form of a hemiarthroplasty is often performed.

Intertrochanteric fracture

The blood supply to the femoral head is intact and these fractures can be internally fixed. Provided the fracture pattern is suitable these are usually fixed with a DHS.

Subtrochanteric fractures

The fracture pattern is usually unsuitable for DHS fixation and an intramedullary nail is needed.

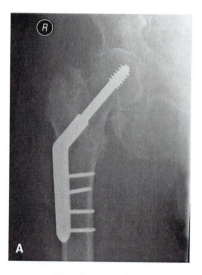

FIGURE 5.12 (a) Radiographs of a dynamic hip screw, (b) hemiarthroplasty and (c) intramedullary nail.

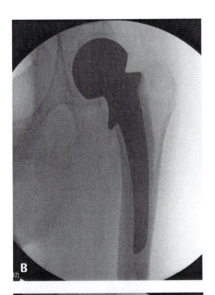

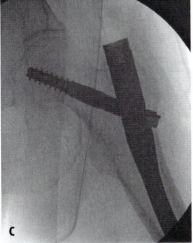

Femoral shaft fractures

Presentation

Femoral shaft fractures usually result from high-energy trauma and patients therefore usually present as a trauma call. If your registrar is not present at the trauma call, then you should inform them of this injury immediately

Assessment and management

Femoral shaft fractures are often associated with extensive blood loss. These fractures should therefore be identified in a primary survey.

Following the basics of resuscitation, if a femoral fracture is suspected then you need to ensure that a splint is applied. There are many different splints available, but essentially it is a device that applies a degree of traction and stabilisation to the limb, which helps to tamponade any blood loss. Urinary catheterisation is essential, unless contraindicated, in order to monitor the volaemic status of the patient.

Splints are temporary measures that can only be applied for short periods of time due to pressure areas and possible tissue necrosis occurring around attachment areas. The femur needs to be definitively stabilised as soon as possible. If the patient is haemodynamically unstable, this needs to be performed as an emergency procedure. A stable patient can be placed in skin traction and definitive stabilisation performed within 24 hours. In adults, stabilisation of the femoral shaft fracture is usually achieved with an intramedullary nail. In children, however, in order to avoid breaching the growth plate, intramedullary nails are normally avoided. Stabilisation is achieved with flexible intramedullary C-nails or open reduction and internal fixation.

Tibial plateau fractures

Tibial plateau fractures are intra-articular fractures of the proximal tibia. The initial management of these injuries from your point of view is straightforward. The complexity lies within the pre-operative planning and definitive management. In order to sustain a tibial plateau fracture a varus- or valgus-deforming force is applied to the knee in combination with axial loading. Lateral tibial plateau fractures are more common than medial plateau fractures.

Clinical assessment

History

It is important that you elicit whether the mechanism of injury is low- or high-energy trauma, as high-energy trauma is associated with an increased risk of complications. Age, co-morbidities, functional ability and social circumstances must be known, as this guides management decisions.

Examination

The examination of tibial plateau fractures is aimed at identifying the complications that are more often associated with high-energy injuries.

- ➲ Vascular compromise – this is very rare. The trifurcation of the popliteal artery is tethered posteriorly and is at risk. If vascular compromise is suspected, then immediate assessment by the vascular surgeons is needed.
- ➲ Neurological injury – the common peroneal nerve is tethered laterally as it winds around the fibular neck and is at risk in tibial plateau fractures. If you identify a nerve palsy, this should be documented but does not require emergency management.

⊃ Compartment syndrome – it is essential that you recognise the possibility of compartment syndrome occurring with tibial plateau fractures and examine for it.

Management

Provided that there are no complications, the initial management of tibial plateau fractures is easy. The fracture needs to be immobilised in a long leg cast and admitted for compartment syndrome observation and further investigations in order to plan definitive treatment.

Schatzker classification

Type I – split-type fracture within the lateral tibial plateau.

Type II – split fracture of the lateral plateau with depressed articular surface.

Type III – depression fracture of the lateral articular surface.

Type IV – medial plateau fracture.

Type V – fractures of the medial and lateral tibial plateaus.

Type VI – tibial plateau fractures with separation of the metaphysis from diaphysis.

The Schatzker classifation is important because it guides management decisions. Tibial plateau fractures are classified from Type I to VI with injury severity and management difficulty increasing accordingly.

A CT scan is usually needed to delineate the fracture pattern in order to plan definitive treatment, the goal of which is always to achieve a congruent joint surface.

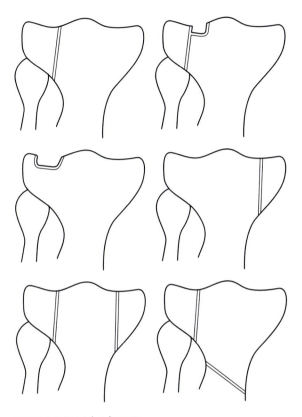

FIGURES 5.13–5.18 Schatzker I–VI.

Schatzker I fractures are often managed conservatively with a period of immobilisation and non-weight bearing.

If there is disruption of the articular surface, then this will need to be restored through open reduction internal fixation in order to reduce the risk of post-operative arthritis.

Ankle fractures

Ankle fractures are common injuries and you will be asked for your 'expert orthopaedic opinion' on many X-rays by the A&E department. Provided you know some basic anatomy and a few simple principles, then managing ankle fractures safely is very straightforward.

Basic ankle anatomy and mechanics

The ankle is a complex hinge joint consisting of articulations between the distal tibia and fibula and the talus. It is stabilised by many ligaments.

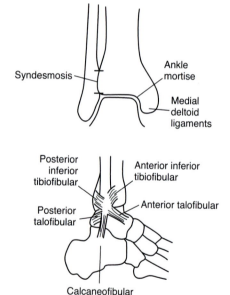

FIGURE 5.19 The complexities of ankle stability.

The distal tibial articular surface together with the medial and lateral malleoli form the mortise. This is a constrained articulation with the talus.

The distal tibiofibular joint is a fibrous joint that is held together by the syndesmosis. This is composed of four different ligaments: anterior inferior tibiofibular, transverse tibiofibular, interosseus membrane and posterior inferior tibiofibular ligament.

Medial support to the ankle is provided by the bony medial malleolus and the large deltoid ligament.

Lateral support is provided by the distal fibula and the fibular collateral ligament, which is made up of three separate ligaments: anterior talofibular, posterior talofibular and calcaneofibular ligaments.

The mortise must be congruent to ensure that the talus moves normally within the ankle joint. If the mortise is disrupted, then the ankle is unstable and the talus will not articulate normally resulting in early degenerative disease.

The most common site for fractures is the lateral malleolus. A medial malleolar fracture in combination with a lateral malleolus fracture is a **bimalleolar** ankle fracture. A **trimalleolar** ankle fracture pattern is a combination of lateral malleolar, medial malleolar and posterior malleolar (the posterior part of the distal tibial articular surface) fractures. In both bimalleolar and trimalleolar ankle fracture patterns the ankle has lost both its medial and lateral support and is therefore inherently unstable.

History

The mechanism of injury will give a clue to the underlying fracture pattern. Age, co-morbidities (particularly diabetes, steroid use and smoking), functional demand and social circumstances are important, as these may influence management decisions.

Examination

Assess the swelling and neurovascular status. Examine for medial and lateral tenderness. Bony tenderness must be assessed for along the entire length of the fibula (remember Maisonneuve injury). On the medial side, you must assess bony and soft-tissue tenderness. Medial soft tissue tenderness may suggest underlying ligament rupture, which if combined with a lateral malleolus fracture may result in an unstable ankle.

Any patient presenting to the emergency department with a deformed, injured ankle must be assumed to have a fracture/dislocation. This requires emergency management, as the blood supply to the foot is at risk. The neurovascular status of the limb should be assessed and the ankle needs to be reduced as an emergency procedure to prevent further compromise to the blood supply and overlying skin.

Emergency reduction of the ankle should not be delayed for X-ray. Radiographs of a fracture/dislocated ankle indicate severe mismanagement and should never be seen.

Reduction of this injury is basic first aid management and should be performed by the A&E team. Unfortunately this is not always the case and it may be left to you. Reduction must be done in the resus room. Sedation, analgesia and monitoring need to be provided. Your only job is to reduce the ankle. Once the patient is safely sedated you can manipulate the ankle. Basically you need to get the ankle looking a normal shape. In order to do this you will need to reverse the deforming forces. Usually this means applying traction, internal rotation and inversion. You will need someone to apply counter-traction and someone to apply a cast. Neurovascular status must be re-assessed post-manipulation.

Interpreting ankle X-rays

It is important that you get a true mortise view (foot 15 degrees internal rotation) and lateral radiographs.

If you suspect a high fibular fracture, clinically you will need to see full tib/fib views.

On the Mortise view, assess for:

- ⮑ fractures of the lateral and/or medial malleolus
- ⮑ congruency of the mortise – i.e. is the distance between the talus and the tibial and fibular articular surfaces equal at all points
- ⮑ talar shift or talar tilt
- ⮑ widening of the distal tibiofibular joint.

On the lateral view:

- ⮑ fractures of the fibular – in particular Weber B fractures, which are not seen on the mortise view
- ⮑ posterior malleolus fractures.

If you see widening of the distal tibiofibular joint, disturbance of the ankle mortise and/or talar shift without any evidence of fractures, you must order full tib/fib views to look for a high fibular Weber C fracture.

Classification

The **Weber** classification is the most commonly used classification system. This is a simple system that directly informs management of the fracture. The Weber system uses the lateral malleolus only.

Weber A: this is a fracture of the lateral malleolus below the level of the syndesmosis. It is usually an avulsion fracture as a result of an inversion type injury. The mortise usually remains congruent and the ankle is stable.

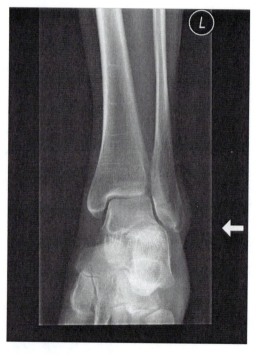

FIGURE 5.20 Weber A fracture of the ankle.

Weber B: this is a fracture that begins at the level of the syndesmosis and may extend more proximally. It is an oblique/spiral fracture pattern, which usually results from an eversion/supination mechanism. The syndesmosis is usually intact. The mortise may or may not be congruent and the ankle may or may not be stable.

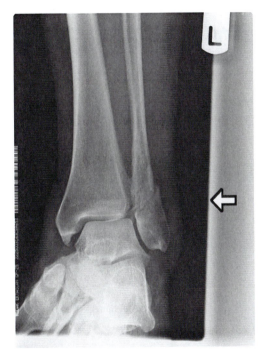

FIGURE 5.21 Weber B fracture of the ankle.

Weber C: this fracture is above the syndesmosis. An eversion/pronation/external rotation force propagates through the ankle, rupturing the syndesotic ligaments and exiting in a fibular fracture above the syndesmosis. The mortise is disrupted and the ankle is unstable. Note that the fibula can be fractured anywhere above the syndesmosis – a high fibula fracture is called a Maisonneuve fracture.

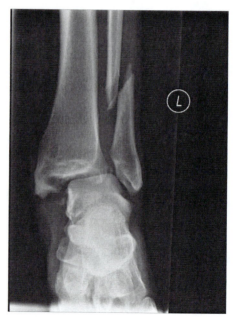

FIGURE 5.22 Weber C fracture of the ankle.

Management

Weber A fractures

These are usually undisplaced or minimally displaced and the ankle is stable. They can therefore be managed non-operatively. Apply a backslab or split cast and re-X-ray in cast to check the fracture hasn't moved. If the position remains the same, then send the patient home non–weight bearing with a 1-week fracture clinic follow-up, X-ray on arrival.

Weber B fractures

These may be managed conservatively or operatively depending on the congruency of the ankle mortise and stability of the fracture.

A Weber B fracture with congruent ankle mortise will be managed conservatively in a backslab or split cast. After application of the cast, you need to repeat the X-ray to check for any loss of position. If the mortise remains congruent, you can send the patient home non–weight bearing. They will need 1-week fracture clinic follow-up, X-ray on arrival.

Displaced Weber B fractures with disruption of ankle mortise and/or talar shift/tilt will need open reduction internal fixation (ORIF). It is often difficult to operate on these early due to swelling and/or theatre availability. Therefore it is important that the ankle is in a safe position, i.e. the mortise is reduced. This will allow the swelling to settle.

In order to reduce the ankle mortise, you will need to manipulate the ankle in the same way as described for fracture/dislocations. A post-manipulation X-ray must be performed, and if this is satisfactory, then the patient should be admitted for high elevation. A swell check will be performed on day 3/4 and if it is safe to operate then ORIF will be performed on the next available trauma list.

Weber C fractures

These almost always need surgical fixation. Manipulate the ankle to reduce the mortise if necessary, place in backslab or split cast and admit for high elevation. ORIF will be performed when the swelling has settled.

Arm fractures and dislocations

Proximal humeral fractures

These fractures are commonly around the surgical neck of the humerus and can involve the greater or lesser tuberosity. The number of fracture fragments should be documented and the patient placed into a collar and cuff. Operative fixation is indicated when the greater tuberosity fracture fragment is displaced by greater than 1 cm or angulated by more than 45 degrees.

Humeral shaft fractures

These are common fractures in the elderly. Assessment of patients needs to include assessment of the radial nerve (motor–wrist drop and sensory), as this can be damaged in these type of fractures due to its passage in the spiral groove on the posterior aspect of the humeral shaft.

These fractures are often treated non-operatively in a collar and cuff, as up to 45 degrees angulation and some shortening can be accepted with no reduction in function.

Shoulder dislocations

These can be anterior (commonest) or posterior. If dislocation cannot be excluded on AP or lateral radiographs, axillary view radiograph (radiograph of the glenohumeral joint with the arm abducted) or a CT scan should be performed.

Anterior dislocations can be reduced with:

- ➲ Kocher's manoeuvre – traction is applied and the shoulder is abducted and externally rotated. The shoulder is then adducted and internally rotated to reduce the dislocation
- ➲ Hippocratic method – with the patient lying down, traction is applied in the line of the body along with counter

traction (commonly a sheet under the axilla being pulled towards the head by an assistant).

Posterior dislocations are often more difficult to reduce and cannot be reduced by Kocher's technique. These dislocations often require operative reduction.

Fracture-dislocations – the dislocation still needs to be reduced emergently in ED prior to any consideration of operative fixation.

Confirmation of reduction should be made with radiographs.

Clavicle fractures

These are common fractures and often involve the mid shaft or the distal third of the clavicle. Initial management should be with broad arm sling. Patients can often be discharged home with fracture clinic follow-up or contact details taken for future management.

Clavicle fractures that often require operative fixation (excluding open fractures) are:

- ➲ displaced high-energy (e.g. biking injures, road traffic accidents) injuries
- ➲ distal third displaced fractures (as have a slightly increased risk of non-union).

Forearm fractures and dislocations

Wrist fractures

These are the commonest type of fractures presenting to hospitals. Fractures are described with regards to:

- angulation (volar or dorsal) – normal wrist is angulated 11 degrees volarly
- shortening (height of distal radius should be level with distal ulna)
- radial inclination (angulation of distal radius on AP radiograph) – normal inclination is 22 degrees.

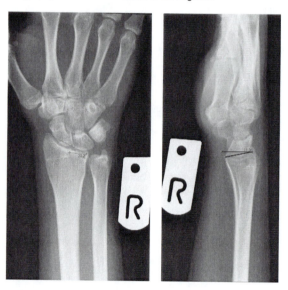

FIGURE 5.23 (a) Normal wrist radiograph – AP, (b) normal wrist radiograph – lateral.

Basic management is to place the wrist into a below-elbow backslab. Patients can often be discharged home with fracture clinic follow-up or contact details taken for future management. Further management can be decided using various factors (excluding open fractures and those with neurovascular compromise which require emergent treatment).

Extra-articular fractures

These generally only require manipulation under the emergency department (ED) with

- ➲ haematoma block (infiltration of local anaesthetic into fracture site)
- ➲ Bier's block (usually performed by ED/anaesthetics)
- ➲ general anaesthetic/sedation.

Intra-articular fractures

These generally require restoration of normal anatomy, which takes the form of operative fixation (exceptions are sometimes made for certain patients and fractures). This is undertaken in theatre by the orthopaedic team with either K-wires or with plate and screw fixation. Patients can be immobilised in a below-elbow backslab and can often be sent home, discussed with the orthopaedic team at the next trauma meeting and booked in for surgery. Very displaced fractures should still be manipulated in ED to reduce the risk of median nerve palsy.

Common eponyms

Colles' fracture – these are fractures that have the classic dinner fork deformity, which were initially described in the 1800s, without radiographs, as a clinical deformity. They are dorsally angulated distal radial fractures.

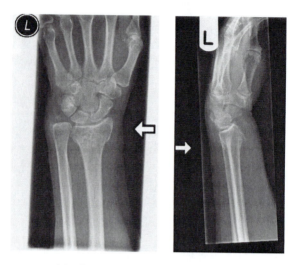

FIGURE 5.24 (a) Colles' fracture – AP, (b) Colles' fracture – lateral.

Smith's fractures – often called reverse Colles' fractures. They are volarly angulated fractures.

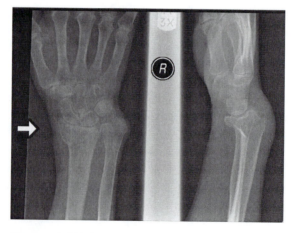

FIGURE 5.25 Smith's fracture.

Radius and ulna fractures (excluding distal radial fractures)

The forearm is a complete ring formed by the radius, ulna, radial head and the distal radius and ulna joint (DRUJ). Like a polo mint, it is difficult to break in just one place. Two parts of the ring are likely to be broken in more than one place and so fractures should be investigated accordingly. These type of fractures often require operative fixation to restore anatomy to full pronation and supination. Basic ED management should start with an above elbow backslab.

Special considerations

- ○ Galeazzi fractures – fractures of the radial shaft with dislocation of the distal radio-ulnar joint. These require operative fixation.
- ○ Monteggia fractures – fractures of the ulna shaft with dislocation of the radial head. These require operative fixation.
- ○ Nightstick fractures – isolated ulna shaft fractures usually resulting from direct trauma. These have a higher risk of non-union, so often require operative fixation.

Olecranon fractures

These often result from indirect trauma and the sudden pull of triceps and brachialis. They result in an intra-articular fracture of the olecranon. Assessment needs to be made of the ability of the patient to extend their elbow against gravity. If they are able to do this, then they can be managed non-operatively in an above elbow cast. Inability to extend the elbow usually requires operative fixation, although exceptions are made for certain, often very elderly patients.

Pathological fractures

These are fractures that occur through areas of weak bone. Most commonly this is through osteoporotic bone but can occur through a bone tumour (benign or malignant), the commonest of which is through a secondary bony metastasis.

If there is any suspicious bony lesion present around the fracture (lytic lesion, sclerotic lesion or cortical thinning), history taking needs to include symptoms of malignancy (weight loss, appetite loss, breast lumps, haematuria, bowel changes, etc.) and history of malignancy along with known metastases. Other bony and joint pain should be documented along with the amount of preceding pain in the fractured bone.

Examination needs to include a thorough examination including breast, abdominal and prostate. Blood tests need to include liver function tests along with a myeloma screen (to include Bence-Jones urinary proteins) as well as routine tests. Chest radiograph should be obtained along with full-length radiographs of the affected bone to check for other lesions.

If primary pathology is unknown, then histological diagnosis needs to be obtained and often referral to a specialist bone tumour centre can be undertaken.

Pathological fractures almost always need operative fixation due to an extremely high risk of severe pain, loss of function and non-union. After operative fixation, radiotherapy may be undertaken (once operative wounds have healed).

Occasionally, patients are referred with painful bony metastases without fracture. Treatment of these is more complex and a decision needs to be taken whether to prophylactically fix these bones to prevent pathological fracture occurring. The Mirels scoring system can be used to help predict the likelihood of fracture. If a patient scores 8 or higher, they are at imminent risk of fracture and so require prophylactic fixation and discussion with a senior colleague is advised.

THE MIRELS SCORING SYSTEM.

Points scored	Site	Size	Type of lesion	Pain
1	Upper limb	<$\frac{1}{3}$ of bone diameter	Blastic (increase signal)	Mild
2	Lower limb	$\frac{1}{3}$–$\frac{2}{3}$	Mixed lytic and blastic	Moderate
3	Proximal femur	>$\frac{2}{3}$	Lytic	Functional (i.e. on walking)

Source: Mirels H. Metastatic disease in long bones. A proposed scoring system for diagnosing impending pathological fractures. *Clin Orthop Relat Res.* 1989 Dec; (249): 256–64.

Septic arthritis

As the orthopaedic SHO on call, you will take many referrals about patients with a possible septic arthritis from GPs, A&E and the wards. A septic arthritis in a native joint is relatively straightforward to diagnose and manage. However, infected prosthetic joints are more difficult to deal with.

Septic arthritis in native joints

Presentation

There is a short history (usually no longer than 72 hours) of progressively worsening joint pain, swelling and loss of function. The patient may or may not be systemically unwell.

On examination features of systemic sepsis must be identified. The joint itself is often hot, swollen and tender. The key feature of a septic joint is a painful, reduced range of movement. Usually the joint can only move through a few degrees and this is very painful.

Investigations

Full blood count, U&E and CRP must be done in order to assess inflammatory markers and also to identify dehydration, etc. as a marker of the septic process. The joint should also be X-rayed in order to identify occult trauma and/or degenerative disease.

If the history, examination and blood findings are suggestive of a septic arthritis, then the definitive investigation is a joint aspirate. This should be performed under aseptic conditions. Once obtained, the samples should be sent to microbiology for urgent analysis. You will most commonly be referred a possibly septic knee, so it is useful to be able to aspirate this joint.

You need to be careful and have a higher index of suspicion

in patients with depressed immune function, as septic joints in these patients can present with a more insidious history and less impressive examination and investigation findings.

> **Knee aspiration**
>
> This must be done under aseptic conditions. It is useful to mark your entry point prior to preparing the skin. The classic entry point used to aspirate the knee is just under the lateral border of the patella in order to get into the patellofemoral joint space. Try to avoid using local anaesthetic prior to the procedure, as this then becomes two needles instead of one and the LA itself is often painful.Once the knee is appropriately prepared it should be aspirated using your planned landmarks. A white needle should be used, as the aspirate is often too thick for smaller needles. The knee should be drained dry if possible, as this often relieves discomfort in the non-septic joints. Once you have gained the aspirate, this must be placed in a sterile pot and sent to microbiology immediately.

Management

The patient should be kept nil by mouth from the time of referral to yourself. A systemically unwell patient who has a good history and examination for septic arthritis should be fluid resuscitated and started on the appropriate IV antibiotics once the joint aspirate has been taken. Early referral to ITU should be considered in the sick patient.

Antibiotics should never be started before the aspirate has been taken. If you don't feel confident taking the sample, you need to tell your registrar early so they can take it urgently before antibiotics are started. Antibiotics should be given according to local policy. If you are uncertain and you need to give something quickly, then IV co-amoxiclav or a combination of benzylpenicillin and flucloxacillin can be given. If the aspirate confirms the presence of organisms, then the patient will need a joint washout in theatre as an emergency.

Differential diagnosis

A number of other conditions can have similar presenting features to an infected joint.

Cellulitis over a joint can present as a red, hot, swollen joint. However, there is usually less reduction in the joint range of movement compared with a septic joint. You should never aspirate a joint through an area of cellulitis, as it risks introducing infection.

Gout has a very similar presentation and examination finding to septic arthritis. The two conditions are often only distinguished through joint aspiration. With gout no organisms are present in the aspirate and crystals may be seen.

Acute exacerbations of osteoarthritis can present in a similar way to septic joints, but the aspirate will have an absence of organisms.

Pre-patella and olecranon bursitis are often referred as possible septic arthritis of the underlying joint. In the case of bursitis, a fluctuant and often tender bursa is seen and the underlying joint moves more freely than would be expected in a septic joint. Never aspirate a joint in the presence of an infected/inflamed bursa.

Septic prosthetic joints

Infected prosthetic joints often present with a longer history and less impressive examination and investigation findings compared with infected native joints.

History

You need to know how long the joint has been in and ideally who put it in. Previous wound or deep infections must be identified. Ongoing pain and disability related to prosthesis must be asked about.

Examination and investigations

There is often a less impressive reduction in range of movement compared with infected native joints. Inflammatory markers are often less significantly raised. If an infected prosthesis is suspected, then the patient should be admitted and undergo aspiration under sterile conditions in the operating theatre. Joint aspiration should never be done on the ward or in A&E.

Management

Antibiotics should never be given before the joint is aspirated. If the patient is systemically well, the joint aspirate can be performed on the next available list. In a systemically unwell patient emergency aspiration in theatre should be performed proceeding to washout as indicated.

Tendon injuries

These occur after trauma and are most often associated with an open laceration over the tendon. Assessment of the flexor or extensor tendon should be made with movement assessed at the metacarpal-phalangeal joint (MCPJ), proximal interphalangeal joint (PIPJ) and distal interphalangeal joint (DIPJ) with movement of each assessed in isolation (i.e. with other joints in the hand stabilised).

Treatment should commence with thorough washout of the wound and a dose of intravenous antibiotics if there is any suspicion of infection. Local anaesthetic may need to be locally infiltrated and often in the form of a ring block. A ring block is performed by infiltrating local anaesthetic (*without* adrenaline) around the base of the digit to anaesthetise the whole digit.

Tendon ruptures should be repaired as soon as possible although delay of the repair (within 7 days) does not compromise outcome. Repair should be performed in theatre along with thorough washout. Patients can often be sent home pending surgery in a splint or plaster.

Mallet finger

Mallet finger is damage to the extensor tendon at its insertion into the distal phalynx. This results in patients being unable to extend their DIPJ and is often a closed injury. Radiograph needs to be obtained to assess if fracture of the base of the distal phalynx is present.

Mallet fingers can be managed in a mallet splint, holding the distal phalynx in extension, if there is no fracture of the distal phalynx present or if the fracture involves less than 50% of the joint surface of the DIPJ. Fractures greater than 50% of the articular surface require operative fixation.

Chapter 6

TRAUMA

Tom König

Trauma management

An Advanced Trauma Life Support (ATLS) provider course qualification is a good start when gaining experience of trauma management. The make up of a trauma team varies between hospitals and with it the role you may have to play. If you are in a major trauma centre (MTC), the support may be quite different to that in a trauma centre (TC). As a surgical SHO/FY2, your role may be to only assess circulation and 'feel the belly' or you may be responsible for assessing and treating any problems that are encountered during the primary survey and later secondary survey. What should always be at the back of your mind or indeed at the front, are those injuries and pathologies that will require a 'surgical' procedure or intervention that either you or a senior will have to undertake. You may find yourself the only 'surgeon' on the team. It is important that if you feel out of your depth or the patient is sick and requires immediate life-saving surgery that you call for senior help early. This may also involve alerting the operating theatre or interventional radiology suite.

Mechanism of injury

A lot of information can be gained by having an understanding of mechanism of injury. The faster a car was travelling, the greater the height from which someone has fallen or the heavier the lorry that has driven over someone, the greater the inevitable injury burden. If someone has injuries to the head, chest and lower limbs then go looking for the injury to the abdomen. Assume everything is broken until proven otherwise.

Penetrating trauma patients who are in shock are bleeding and require immediate surgery. Be wary of some fairly trivial sounding mechanisms – handlebar injuries to the abdomen in children are well recognised to cause serious hepatic or splenic injuries.

Investigations

The typical imaging modalities used in trauma include plain radiographs of the chest, pelvis and C-spine. CT scanning is being used more readily and it is important that you try to view the images as quickly as possible with a radiologist who will issue a formal report. Focused Assessment by Sonography in Trauma (FAST) is being used to look for pneumothoraces, pericardial effusion (blood) and tamponade and free intraperitoneal fluid (blood). It is quick and easy but operator dependent. It is best at ruling in than it is at ruling out (i.e. someone who is shocked, has a 'seatbelt sign' across their abdomen and is peritonitic has blood in their belly even if the USS is 'negative'). FAST has generally superseded diagnostic peritoneal lavage (DPL) in looking for peritoneal blood. DPL is invasive and is not without its own complications. DPL is after all, not hugely different to laparoscopic port placement and so won't become a procedure surgeons will forget.

Primary survey

The primary survey is, as its name suggests, the first part of the assessment and management of a trauma patient. It follows the ABC approach. In the military, due to the nature of the injuries seen, catastrophic haemorrhage control comes first.

ABC

In some circumstances it may be possible to carry out all aspects of the primary survey at the same time. If not, then work through them sequentially. If life-threatening problems are found, then these should be treated as quickly as possible before moving on. If someone is able to answer the simple question, 'Hello, what's your name?', then you know that they are protecting their airway, breathing (phonating) and have a blood pressure to perfuse their brain. Job done, you may say!

Airway

This is often the domain of the anaesthetist to assess and secure if the patient is unable to protect their own airway. Various methods of improving the integrity of the airway exist and include: the jaw thrust, nasopharyngeal airways, oropharyngeal airways and laryngeal mask airway. The cuffed endotracheal tube is the definitive airway and often requires a general anaesthetic. If the intubation is unsuccessful or the patient has significant airway burns, then surgical cricothyroidotomy may be required. You may not be able to turn and ask your friendly ENT surgeon if they would oblige, so be familiar with the anatomy and the procedure. In essence, make a transverse incision through the skin over the cricothyroid membrane, open it and keep it open, pass a bougie and railroad an endotracheal tube over it.

Breathing

Assessment of the chest involves inspection, palpation, percussion and auscultation (nothing new there). Changes in any should raise your suspicion that there is underlying pathology. Count the respiratory rate, look for symmetry, feel every rib for fractures and subcutaneous surgical emphysema. Absent sounds or wheeze mean there is lung collapse and a pneumothorax. Think about mechanism and history. A driver of a car hit from the side will have rib fractures on the right. Significant flail segments will overlay a lung injury that may require drainage and advanced analgesia or intubation to maintain oxygenation.

A simple pneumothorax may be left alone or require drainage if large. Tension pneumothorax is a pneumothorax with cardiovascular collapse. Drain the air quickly to allow the right heart to fill again and restore cardiac ouput. Stick a large needle in the mid-clavicular line, second intercostal (IC) space or in the fourth IC space anterior axillary line (the thinnest part of the chest and where you'll then place a large-bore 32 Fr intercostal drain).

If the chest radiograph shows a 'white out' and the chest is tender and dull to percussion with reduced breath sounds, suspect a haemothorax. Drainage is often the only treatment required. Local anaesthetic infiltration or intravenous analgesia with ketamine aid insertion. The drain doesn't need to cross the midline, so place it carefully: anterior and apically for air, basally to drain blood. Ask the patient to take a deep breath and watch for 'swinging and bubbling', denoting correct placement and effective treatment. Suture it in place so it doesn't come out.

If the drainage bottle fills immediately and the bleeding continues, then the underlying injury is more serious. Call for help from someone who can fix the problem (trauma surgeon or cardiothoracic surgeon), resuscitate the patient (often with blood and blood products), alert theatres and get ready to move. Clamping the drain tube just keeps the blood in the chest; this patient may well be coagulopathic, so tamponading the chest is unlikely. Resuscitating the patient will buy you time, especially if you have to transfer the patient to another hospital. If the patient arrests, then thoracotomy may be required to control the pleural, great vessel or cardiac source of bleeding.

Cardiac tamponade is a simple injury to both die from and

to treat. A myocardial injury (mostly the result of stabbing injury to the anterior right ventricle) fills the pericardial space with blood, reduces right heart filling, which subsequently causes reduced cardiac output and eventually cardiac arrest. Needle pericardiocentesis is unreliable, can cause myocardial injury and formed clot evacuation is nigh on impossible. Left anterolateral, or 'clamshell' thoracotomy allows quick access to the heart and lungs, permits rapid opening of the pericardium before temporary control or definitive suture of the myocardial wound. This is easy to say if you've done it or seen it a few times; the difficulties are often in the decision to undertake the procedure in the first place. The patient will die if you do nothing. Thoracotomy is a required training competency of every general surgical registrar.

Circulation

There are various classes of shock depending on the heart rate, blood pressure and level of consciousness, etc. Thinking about the volume of blood loss will guide you when you resuscitate patients with what fluid you'll use. Look at the patient. Are they pale, sweaty, lethargic, cold and are they perfusing their extremities? If a patient is not perfusing their big toe, then they're shut down and relying on their sympathetic response to maintain blood pressure – a bad sign! Do you want to spend a long time with this patient in a CT scanner while they continue to bleed their own blood that you are replacing with saline, which neither clots nor carries oxygen, while being observed to death? Think about mechanism again – deceleration injuries can result in aortic transection distal to the ligamentum arteriosum, splenic injury or mesenteric injury. Again, with a high index of suspicion, go looking for the injuries and you'll either find them or confidently exclude them and reduce the missed injury rate.

Large-bore peripheral or central intravenous access is key. Take blood for a blood gas, clotting and group and save. Ongoing bleeding from penetrating wounds requires surgery to control or restore integrity. Think about temporary measures at controlling bleeding that you can do in the resuscitation room. Don't be tempted to 'cover and peek' constantly. Put a dressing on, press hard, elevate if you can and wait. Early administration of local anaesthetic with adrenaline early both reduces pain and stops bleeding. Put some large sutures in a wound to reduce blood loss. Larger vessel injuries may require proximal tourniquet (either military type or pneumatic) placement. In this case the patient should probably be in an operating theatre sooner rather than later.

Truncal bleeding or bleeding from junctional areas that are not amenable to compression need surgery as soon as possible. Injuries to the groin or neck can be pressed on, or wound tracks filled with topical haemostatic agents or Foley catheters but these efforts should not prolong the time to theatre. Modern imaging is all well and good, but don't forget that the human eye is also capable of revealing a lot of information. Surgeons would much rather do a laparotomy or vascular repair in a well-lit and well-stocked operating theatre, so go there ASAP.

Disability

This is traditionally the assessment of the Glasgow Coma Score to document the level of consciousness. Best eye opening, verbal response and motor response to stimuli are measured with a minimum score of 3 and maximum of 15. A score lower than 8/15 implies that definitive airway control is required. Conscious level may fall with blood loss but often implies head injury.

Other surgical procedures

Patients suffering traumatic injury present in a wide variety of ways. Severe burns may require escharotomy to permit adequate ventilation or to prevent compartment syndrome in extremities.

Partial/non-complete amputation may require completion in the resuscitation room.

Traumatic cardiac arrest in a pregnant woman requires immediate caesarean section to deliver the foetus and reduce the cardiovascular workload of the mother. This intervention is obviously not for the faint hearted but any surgical procedure for those in extremis should be considered, especially for those who will undoubtedly die without intervention. The team leader may suggest a surgical intervention and turn to you to either carry it out or to assist them in the process.

Now it's time to move onto the secondary survey. This may not be your role in the team but if you can do it, it expedites the patient's journey through the emergency department onto the ward. Make sure you document everything you have done and record the trauma call and surgical procedures carried out for your logbook.

The trauma laparotomy

Now you've done all that needs to be done in the resuscitation room and the patient may even have been well enough to go through the CT scanner! Some injured organs are now more likely to be treated conservatively. They even include high-grade liver and spleen injuries. They need to be closely observed and ideally the same person should re-examine the abdomen. Bleeding from these organs may also be embolised radiologically.

For those patients that are unstable, the trauma laparotomy is the next step. Damage control surgery (DCS) is an abbreviated procedure which aims to restore physiology, as opposed to anatomy. It's used for those patients who are cold, coagulopathic, acidotic and who present in extremis. They often require a massive transfusion and tranexamic acid, and will be going to the intensive care unit after surgery. Most hospitals have their own massive transfusion protocol, which will need to be activated. The goal of trauma laparotomies is control of bleeding, normally initially with packing.

Chapter 7

THE WARDS

Shelly Griffiths and
Emma Noble

Ward cover

Your day and night shifts will continue to be plagued by countless calls to attend unwell ward patients. Effective prioritisation is key. This chapter aims to give you a guide on how to manage unwell ward patients. At all times though, remember your ALS principles, and if you ever feel out of control in a situation, call your senior sooner rather than later. However stupid you may feel for calling, you will feel worse if your inaction has adverse consequences.

Securing the **airway** is always the first priority. If you feel an airway is at risk, this is the time for a medical emergency or arrest call. Don't forget basic adjuncts and laryngeal mask airways if you're really stuck.

Common causes of tachypnoea in surgical patients:
- pain
- anxiety
- volume depletion (including anaemia)
- infection (systemic as well as pulmonary)
- acute cardiac event
- pulmonary causes (PE, infection, basal atelectasis).

During your assessment of **breathing** you may start to pick up abnormalities that you can deal with, such as an abnormal respiratory rate or low oxygen saturations. If so, supply supplemental oxygen. Tachypnoea may have several causes, and your ongoing assessment will help distinguish between them. A low respiratory rate in the surgical inpatient is often due to opiate toxicity. If this is the case, give naloxone. Remember that the half-life of naloxone is less than that of morphine, and repeat doses may be required. Don't forget to stop or reduce their opiate prescription!

Low oxygen saturations may themselves be the result of any cause of an abnormal respiratory rate, and may be the result of something very basic such as patient position. Give oxygen. There is still some controversy around giving high-flow oxygen to patients with COPD who may depend on their hypoxic drive, and teaching on this subject tends to leave students confused. However, hypoxia will kill much faster than hypercapnoea. To avoid problems, continually re-assess the patient after administering treatment. If a patient worsens with increased oxygen, this is a sign that more controlled oxygen delivery or even respiratory assistance with non-invasive ventilation may be required. Any patient with an abnormality picked up during your assessment of breathing (except the very clear opiate toxicity with a good response to naloxone) will need a chest radiograph and an arterial blood gas (ABG). An ABG is arguably the most useful test in any acutely unwell patient, and will give you a huge amount of information in just a few minutes.

The assessment of **circulation** is key in the surgical patient, and much of it is gained from simply looking at the patient. Observation charts may demonstrate a slow deteriorioration or sudden change with increasing tachycardia and hypoten-sion. The speed of decline may help with your diagnosis. Are they shut down peripherally or do they have a hyperdynamic circulation? This simple observation will tell you a lot about what is going on. You need to remember the different causes of shock and work out which one is affecting your patient. If somebody is hypotensive, you need to assess what impact this is having. Are they still cerebrating and perfusing their kidneys? Give a fluid bolus and remember to review the response to this.

> ### The 'C's of post-operative pyrexia
> - Chest
> - Catheter
> - Cannula/CVP line
> - Calves (DVT)
> - Cut (wound infection)
> - Collection

Urine output should be reviewed as part of your assessment of circulation, and if the patient is unwell a catheter should be sited (attached to a urometer) to allow accurate assessment. Often though, you will be called to an otherwise seemingly well patient with a low urine output. Remember that an acceptable urine output is a weight-based measurement. An output of 0.5 mL/kg/hr is fine – make sure you think about the size of the patient when assessing their urine output. The nursing staff will normally have tried the basics, like flushing the catheter, but if they haven't, make sure you do. If there is a genuine anuria or oliguria, you need to check renal function and, if deranged, assess the acid–base balance of the patient with an ABG.

Acute kidney injury secondary to volume depletion is unfortunately common in the surgical patient. Fluid replacement must be tailored to the individual patient, based on their co-morbidities. Boluses of 250 mL of crystalloid are often appropriate. Again, remember to monitor the response.

Post-operative **pyrexia** has a number of potential causes. The length of time that has lapsed since the operation may give you some clues as to the cause, though this is a very rough guide and should not replace your clinical assessment:

- 24 hours – atelectasis
- 24–48 hours – atelectasis, lower respiratory tract infection
- Day 3+ – urinary tract infection
- Day 5+ – wound infection
- Day 7+ – DVT.

Of course, not all of your patients will be post-operative, and the primary or admitting pathology may be to blame, such as diverticulitis. In addition to thinking about the cause, take a full set of bloods (to include inflammatory markers and renal function) and blood cultures. Some departments advocate two sets of cultures from different venepuncture sites to try and increase pick-up rates of bacteraemia. Think about antibiotics – do they need to be started? This may not always be indicated, though if somebody is septic, antibiotics must not be delayed whilst hunting for a cause. If already on antibiotics, they may need to be altered, and microbiology advice will often be needed.

> **Common causes of chest pain:**
> - acute cardiac event
> - PE
> - LRTI
> - reflux
> - musculoskeletal.

Another common problem will be the surgical patient with **chest pain**. There is no difference between managing the surgical patient and any other with chest pain – but remember that a PE is slightly more likely, particularly if they have had pelvic or lower limb surgery or have a malignancy. After assessing the patient's ABC status and starting treatment, obtain an ECG, check bloods (including for a troponin rise with an immediate and a delayed test at 6 hours after the event) and consider if a CTPA is appropriate. If you think the cause is cardiac, a medical opinion is essential.

Another common problem in the surgical inpatient is new onset **atrial fibrillation** (AF). Confirm the presence of this with an ECG. As well as treating the AF itself, you need to think about the cause (most often sepsis). This may be the first subtle sign of a complication such as anastomotic leak, so a cause must be sought. If the patient is compromised and the AF really is new, cardioversion should be considered. If the patient is stable and the AF is fast, you need to think about rate control with either digoxin or a beta-blocker. Medical advice may well be useful.

You may also be called to review **abnormal blood results**, anything from raised inflammatory markers to abnormal electrolytes. In the case of raised inflammatory markers, clinically assess the patient and perform a septic screen (blood cultures, respiratory examination and urinalysis). Start antibiotics if appropriate, but never just for raised inflammatory markers with an unclear source in a systemically well patient. If a patient is anaemic, you must think about why as well as treating it. Transfusion is indicated in any symptomatic patient (regardless of the absolute value). Transfusion based on absolute values alone (normally <8 g/dL) is a bit more controversial, though may be appropriate, particularly in anybody with a history of cardiac disease. With abnormal electrolytes, hospitals often have their own policy which should be followed. Hyperkalaemia is the most common – make sure the result is genuine (i.e. repeat blood electrolytes ensuring the sample is not taken from an arm receiving an infusion) and you have done an ECG (and compared it to an old one). If treatment is needed, make sure you stop any sources of potassium as well!

Escalation of care

There may be occasions where your immense medical skills still leave you with an acutely unwell patient. The question you need to ask yourself is does this patient need urgent surgical intervention or do they require further medical support, normally in the form of a high dependency or intensive treatment unit. Your registrar should be involved at this point. If things are really dire, never delay in putting out a medical emergency call (still an arrest call in some hospitals) or contacting the intensive care unit directly.

If you are going to call for an intensive care review, you need to know what your patient needs that they may be able to offer. Normally this will be in the form of respiratory or cardiovascular support. First though, you have to think about whether an escalation of care is appropriate for your patient. This should not be your decision alone; your registrar and the intensivists themselves will have an opinion. If you know your patient is not suitable for ICU though, it's unfair to call the intensivists to ask them to make that decision for you.

Specialty-specific problems

A lot of problems you will be called to see on the ward will be specific to the specialty a patient has been admitted under or the operation they have had. Some of these problems have already been discussed in the appropriate chapter. It would be impossible to cover all of them here, but the most common are listed below.

Post-operative ileus

This is a functional problem with the bowel, often as a result of handling intra-operatively, but it may occur following surgery to any site of the body. Opiate use and electrolyte abnormalities are causative factors, so make sure they have been assessed. It presents with the standard features of obstruction, and should be managed as such, with an NG tube and IV fluids. Remember though to think of mechanical causes of obstruction which may occur post-operatively. Complications that result in bowel obstruction are varied and can be anything from bowel kinking within a haematoma to a misplaced suture.

Stoma problems

Staff nurses on colorectal wards are normally expert in assessing stomas and will be in contact with you if they suspect a problem. Post-operatively (particularly after emergency surgery) stomas may be very oedematous. This normally settles without intervention, but insertion of a foley catheter into the stoma can sometimes be useful to exclude this as a cause of obstruction. A dusky stoma, though, is more serious, and this ischaemia can make a patient as unwell as any ischaemic bowel. Remember to check an arterial lactate. A return to theatre with re-do of the stoma may well be required. Stomas can prolapse acutely, which will become more difficult to reduce as time progresses. Manual reduction should therefore be attempted (after administration of analgesia), so do not be afraid to handle stomas.

Anastomotic leak

A possible leak is a risk with any primary anastomosis, whether or not it is covered with a defunctioning stoma proximally. Those that aren't covered tend to present more acutely. Emergency cases are at higher risk. A leak classically happens around day 5–7 post-operatively. Systemic features of sepsis, along with abdominal pain, will be present but may be subtle (e.g. a rising CRP/WBC, low-grade pyrexia, tachycardia, new onset AF). Most patients will be well enough for a CT to confirm the diagnosis prior to re-exploration of the abdomen. Work-up as for any acutely unwell patient, and get your registrar involved early.

TURP syndrome

This is pretty rare, but still appears in all the textbooks. It is more likely to present whilst the patient is still in theatre than later on the ward. If it does occur though, you need to act quickly. It is caused by systemic absorption of the irrigation fluid used during TURP and presents with fluid overload and hyponatraemia. Symptoms include confusion (progressing to a reduced level of consciousness), nausea and vomiting. Tachycardia, and initial hypertension followed by hypotension may be seen. The hypotension will not respond to fluid boluses. Careful fluid balance is vital and may necessitate admission to HDU. The sodium normally comes up on its own over time with fluid restriction. Be careful of replacing too rapidly.

Loss of bladder irrigation fluid

You may well be called by the nursing staff due to an imbalance between the amount of fluid put in to irrigate a bladder for haematuria and the amount coming out. Be suspicious of the accuracy of the fluid balance charts, as losses from bypassing catheters or poor record-keeping are normally responsible. The only other explanation would be a perforated bladder, in which case you would be faced with a seriously unwell patient whose problems should be much greater than a fluid chart imbalance.

Tracheostomies

Many juniors are (quite rightly!) nervous around tracheostomies. Nurses on appropriate wards are often much more comfortable and experienced in managing them. However, you may well be called if a tracheostomy becomes blocked or displaced. A spare is often kept at the bedside and simply needs to be quickly replaced. If you are worried, ask the nurse to get an urgent anaesthetic presence whilst you attempt to replace it.

Post-thyroidectomy problems

The most common problem people worry about is the post-operative haematoma resulting in a compromised airway. This is actually pretty uncommon. It will be obvious if it is occurring though; your role is to quickly open the wound on the ward and organise getting the patient back to theatre. Surgeons may use surgical clips to close the wound and will supply a clip remover to accompany the patient to the ward.

The other worry post-thyroidectomy is hypocalcaemia secondary to damage to the parathyroid glands. There is about a 30% risk of this after total or completion thyroidectomy. This may be temporary or permanent. Look for evidence of tetany, and check an ECG. If symptomatic, calcium replacement should be intravenous initially with a later oral replacement (if still indicated).

Post-laryngectomy problems

These may also trouble you. The most common cause of breathing difficulties will be a blocked stoma requiring decrusting. This is normally because of poor humidification and stoma care. After you've cleaned it, make sure humidified air is being used and encourage better care to prevent further calls. A patient with a tracheo-oesophageal puncture for a speech valve will initially have a Foley catheter inserted for feeding. Displacement should be managed with immediate replacement – use a size 12–16G male Foley catheter to prevent closure. The same should be done for a patient with a valve which has fallen out. Finally, remember in an arrest situation that oxygen should go over the stoma and not the nose and mouth and that the anaesthetist will get nowhere attempting to intubate through the mouth!

Drain problems

The leaking or blocked drain is another common call. Drains may be inserted intraoperatively, to deal with post-operative complications or as a primary treatment (e.g. a diverticular abscess). When asked to review a drain firstly make sure you know who put the drain in and why. If placed intra-operatively it is usually to detect haemorrhage but there may be specific instructions on the operation note so check before seeing the patient. If fluid is leaking from the drain site it is usually safe to flush the drain with a small volume of saline to clear any blockages within the tubing. Drains should not be painful, so examine the drain site for signs of infection if pain is the main symptom. Do not forget to examine the whole patient to check for signs that something more serious is going on. If in doubt, leave drains in place until you can check with a senior colleague.

Urethral catheters

These may have been inserted for a variety of reasons, e.g. monitoring of urine output, acute or chronic retention or post prostatic or bladder surgery. As already mentioned, a forceful flush of the catheter may be all that is required to clear a blocked catheter. You may also be called for advice on whether a catheter can be removed. Again, make sure you find out why and when the catheter was inserted and look for any post-operative instructions from the operating note. If the patient is well and has no previous prostate or bladder issues, it may be safe to remove. However, beware the patient who has had a section of bladder resected during colorectal surgery. These catheters need to stay in for at least 2 weeks (or until a contrast study has been done) to decompress the bladder and allow it to heal. Surgical wards are no stranger to the confused elderly patient who forcibly removes their urethral catheter. It is normal to see a small amount of blood after such an occurrence, but re-inserting a catheter may compound a urethral injury. Assess their need for a catheter, and don't be afraid to call a urologist for advice.

Post-operative haematomas

The urgency of management of this depends on the operation that has been performed. Most will be managed conservatively, but there are some situations where you'll need to get a senior decision about taking a patient back to theatre for exploration. This mainly applies to vascular patients and those that have had breast or plastic procedures with flaps which may be at risk. Make sure up-to-date blood tests (group and save, Hb and clotting) have been performed.

Graft occlusion

A newly inserted graft becoming blocked is usually first noticed by the nurses doing their post-operative foot observations when a pulse becomes impalpable or a Doppler signal disappears. The patient may be asymptomatic, especially if they have an epidural in. Assess the foot yourself carefully in the way you always would assess for an ischaemic foot, and you must especially listen with a Doppler probe. Usually the vascular surgeon will draw a cross where the pulse could be felt/heard at the end of the operation. It's absolutely essential to read (and understand!) the operation note so you can get an idea of the plumbing. An ischaemic foot post bypass surgery may need urgent surgery to resurrect the graft. Let the vascular surgeon on call know if there are any concerns about his graft.

Compartment syndrome

Severe increasing pain in the leg within 24 hours of a bypass may be seen if the bypass was done for acute severe ischaemia. The reperfused muscle swells, causing compartment syndrome. More is written about this in Chapter 5, 'Orthopaedics' (see pp. 132–137): it may need urgent fasciotomy.

Index

Entries in **bold** denote figures and tables.